REPACKING FOR GREECE

Repacking for Greece

A Mediterranean Odyssey

Sally Jane Smith

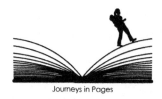

Journeys in Pages

First published by Journeys in Pages, 2024

ISBN 978-0-6456257-2-1 (paperback)
ISBN 978-0-6456257-3-8 (e-book)

Cover design by Andrew Brown of Design for Writers
Internal design by Rebecca Brown of Design for Writers
Author photographs by Mariel Hacking and Adam Hobson

A catalogue record for this book is available from the National Library of Australia

For Adam.
Because living with a writer isn't easy,
but he still seems happy to see me when I return home from my travels.

And for everyone who showed me kindness in Sri Lanka,
especially Aruna, Chamila and their families.

CONTENTS

PREFACE:
UNPACKING FOR GREECE

*R*EPACKING FOR *GREECE* IS a stand-alone travel story, but readers might find it helpful to know what came before.

In Sally's first book, *Unpacking for Greece*, she set out from Australia to Europe to tackle her fear of road travel. With her mum's 1978 travel diary in hand, and the weight of a midlife crisis on her back, she embarked on a quest to reclaim the wanderlust she'd lost in a traumatic bus accident in Sri Lanka.

As she ventured into the heart of the Mediterranean — wandering volatile landscapes, exploring historical sites, pairing books with places and savouring the tastes of Greece — she found it was possible for a clumsy, out-of-shape woman on a budget to experience a life-changing journey.

Sally encountered a memorable cast of characters during her first Greek trip, including a manipulative taxi driver, two tour guides (one inspirational and the other downright creepy), a flirtatious hotelier and a charismatic cat. But her most important companions turned out to be the ones who weren't even there: her sisters — both those in blood and those in spirit — and the enigmatic travel notes left by her mother, who died when Sally was in her twenties.

Greece sparked Sally's tumble into love with her own life again. It also turned her into a writer, when she woke one morning from a dream that she was working on a manuscript about her travels. But when she flew out from Rhodes airport on a marathon fifty-hour return journey to her home in Australia, she had no idea she would be returning to Greek shores any time soon.

Map of Greece

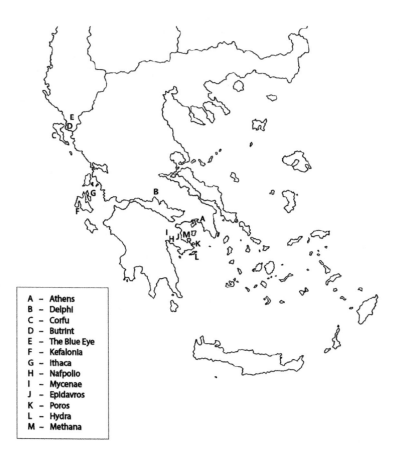

A – Athens
B – Delphi
C – Corfu
D – Butrint
E – The Blue Eye
F – Kefalonia
G – Ithaca
H – Nafpolio
I – Mycenae
J – Epidavros
K – Poros
L – Hydra
M – Methana

BEFORE: MEMORY AND CONSEQUENCE

CHAPTER ONE
REMEMBERING APARTHEID
SOUTH AFRICA

I HAD BEEN PLANNING THE Canadian visit for months. So how did I end up disembarking at Athens International Airport instead, a mere eight months after my life-changing first journey to Greece?

Five days before my scheduled flight to Canada, my passport and air ticket sat ready on a table in my Australian flat. A suitcase lay open in a corner of the room, half filled with a jumble of travel essentials. I was all set to explore Vancouver during the last week of a mild May, before heading up to the Rocky Mountains with my nephew, Christopher.

That's how it was supposed to play out, but the consequences of long-forgotten events threw my careful plans into disarray. To understand the bizarre twist that kept me out of Canada and offered me a second Greek adventure, we'll need to go back in time. A long way back, to the country of my birth in the dying days of apartheid.

~ ~ ~

My parents were kind people who tried to lead good lives. They attended a church that was about as non-racial a place of worship as existed in South Africa at the time, and sought out schools for us that admitted pupils of all races. They made genuine sacrifices to help people in need and raised us to make friends and respect our elders regardless of skin colour.

But, make no mistake, I grew up complicit in — and benefitting from — the institutions of racial oppression.

Imagine, if you will, two teenagers on the half-hour afternoon walk from school to the train station. She's fair-haired and self-conscious about her inability to catch a tan. He's most likely what is termed 'Cape Coloured' in apartheid's endless obsession with racial sub-classifications, although she's never asked. They've been classmates for years and get on well: they banter together during lessons, go to many of the same after-school activities, dance at weekend parties. They both score high marks, just one rung down from the three acknowledged brainiacs in their year. They're not especially close, but she considers him a friend.

Mid-chat, she parrots a gag from a poorly photocopied page that's been handed around school in the way these things were done before the internet gave us memes. It's a weak joke that relies on racial degradation for its humour, but she hasn't given this a thought. She's suppressing a giggle, waiting for his explosive laugh at the punchline.

Instead — to her shock, because she's had the privilege of ignoring the systemic imbalance of power that lurks beneath their friendship — he calls her out.

It's less shameful to pretend that girl wasn't me, but I'm not fooling anybody.

Powerful as this memory is, I have no recollection of my friend's words. But the takeaway message was clear: *It's easy to claim skin colour doesn't matter if you're not the one bleeding because of it.*

Once he had confronted me with the relentless violations of apartheid, it was impossible to let things go. The blinkers were off and, everywhere I turned, I witnessed the brutal underbelly of my soft lifestyle. Before I left high school, I became a political activist.

Let's put that statement in perspective. Yes, there were white heroes in the struggle against racial injustice, both sung and unsung, and I am honoured to know a few. But they were not many, and I was not one of them. Nevertheless, although my role in the uprising was so minor as to fade into insignificance, it was all-consuming for me.

At seventeen, I joined a Cape Youth Congress branch that gathered each week in the crypt of an Anglican church. My mother agreed to ferry me into the city every Sunday evening. With the lack of mindfulness typical of an adolescent, it didn't occur to me what a bother it was for her to drive the forty-kilometre round trip. With hindsight, I suspect that my parents, who were grappling with my decision to leave their faith, hoped the church connection was much more than a convenient venue. But CAYCO wasn't a religious organisation. It acted as a wing of Nelson Mandela's African National Congress Youth League, which had gone into exile when the government banned the ANC in 1960.

Mum continued to cart me to and fro every week until I finished school, got a full-time job in a city bank and, unable to afford a place of my own, moved into Cape Town's YWCA. This communal residence for young women gave me an independence from my family I considered well worth the evening curfews and mandatory weekly religious services. Its location within walking distance of the CAYCO meetings was a valuable bonus.

~ ~ ~

Nelson Mandela's release from prison on 11 February 1990 marked my political coming of age.

Years before emails were commonplace, the summons came through the activist phone network. The YWCA's payphone was tucked behind a staircase, in an uncomfortable nook usually filled with giggling gossip or murmured endearments. This call was to be very different. It was a Saturday, just a few hours before the public announcement that Mandela would walk free the next afternoon, and the voice on the other end of the line was flustered. The caller was working their way through a lengthy phone list, mobilising community activists to help with preparations for a rally to welcome him.

Rumour and conjecture had been running wild for the last eight days. On 2 February, headlines had blazoned out the news of the unbanning of the African National Congress and other organisations that had campaigned against apartheid for decades. From the moment the ban against the ANC was lifted, almost every conversation turned to whether the government would release its most famous political prisoner, and when. This hurried exchange on the YWCA payphone wasn't speculation, though. This time it was real. I signed out of the building for the night, as we would be hard at work until long after my curfew.

Hundreds converged on the University of the Western Cape, *toyi-toying*[1] in a joyous frenzy of celebration while we waited

---

1   The South African *toyi-toyi* is a combination of chanting and dance that expresses defiant protest or, in this case, victorious jubilation. It is not easy to describe without belittling its power, but the song can range from plaintive melody to a militant call and response, and body movements include anything from a shuffling jog that can be sustained over long marches to a high-stepping foot stomp that builds courage in the face of danger.

for our leaders to assign tasks. Many of us were oblivious to the logistical monster they were tackling behind the scenes. While we chanted and danced, they were struggling to confirm a venue for the largest gathering Cape Town had ever seen.

We split into groups, each with a job to do. My team's brief was to replicate a hastily designed pamphlet with a simple message in black on white:

MANDELA SPEAKS
PARADE
SUN 11 FEB 3 PM

I piled paper into a wheezy old photocopier. My friends tackled the results, some with scissors, others using rulers to tear the sheets into careful halves. 'How can we have a revolution,' we joked, 'if we don't have a guillotine?'

Early on Sunday morning, a bunch of CAYCO youth piled into an old VW Kombi minibus draped with the ANC flag. This blatant display was an act of both pride and insurrection; it wasn't long since it had been an imprisonable offence. Fuelled by adrenaline and a couple of hours' sleep, we drove through seaside suburbs, calling out the news until we were hoarse. Our aim was to let all who wanted to welcome this great man — especially Black domestic workers living in the 'servants' quarters' of white households — know they could come to the Parade to hear him speak.

The 'Parade' wasn't a procession; it was a place. The Grand Parade was once Cape Town's main public square, but in 1990 it was just a paved space in front of the historic City Hall building that had been repurposed to house a cramped library and a few municipal services. The square itself was underused, except for the busy kiosks selling takeaway food along one edge.

On that day, the Grand Parade was unrecognisable. My heart soared at the sight of the ANC's green, black and gold colours flying from the City Hall, and the thousands upon thousands of people streaming in from every direction, more than I have ever seen in one place, before or since. But as the hot hours wore on with no sign of Mandela, the crowd grew larger. Thirstier. Angrier.

A confusion of human figures covered every surface, clambering up to every vantage point. The roofs of the kiosks lining the edge of the Grand Parade collapsed from the burden of the bodies they bore, as did the tower that had been set up for the press. People swarmed up tall palm trees and thudded to the ground when sturdy fronds snapped under their weight. I later heard that former United States presidential candidate Jesse Jackson had insisted, against the advice of rally organisers, on riding 'through the people'. Marshals had to pull him and his wife from their vehicle, pass them over the heads of the throng and haul them up to the speakers' balcony. The load of those climbing onto the roof of their abandoned car flattened it.

A hand grasped my shoulder. It belonged to a man who pulled me into a line of marshals and then vanished into the mêlée. Perhaps he chose me for the struggle slogan on my T-shirt. Maybe he simply grabbed whoever was closest. But I was eighteen years old, just three months out of high school and politically aware for not much longer. I had never been a rally marshal and had only a simplistic understanding of what was happening. All I knew was what he hollered into my ear, barely audible above the surrounding din and clamour. People at the front were being crushed, and lives depended on us damming the swelling flood of those desperate to get close to Mandela, to see his face for the first time. For more than two decades, not even a photograph had escaped his prison.

Arms linked with strangers, the fragile chain of marshals staggered under the surging force of the hundred-thousand-strong crowd. We broke apart, then fought to come together, stretching urgent hands out to each other until we could again feel the precarious grip of sweat-slick fingers.

Spittle from angry mouths, scant inches away, flecked my face.

'Where were you at Sharpeville?' A man's voice cracked, mid-yell, on the name of the town where police killed or wounded more than 250 Black South Africans during the 1960 massacre.

'Where were you in '76?' shouted someone else I couldn't see.

They had a point. What right did this little whitey, an incongruous patch in the line of marshals, have to stand in their way on this day of all days? It's not lost on me now that, whatever the circumstances, I was yet another white person telling people of colour what they could or could not do.

Gunfire rang out as gangsters looted nearby shops. I had to choke down my panic. *Are police firing into the crowd?* It had happened before and would again. Without handheld radios or mobile phones, we had no way to find out. All we could do was the job in front of us: hold our thin human line against the shoving ocean of people as best we could.

There was relief when the multitude thinned after the ordeal of so many hours, but there was also a cloud of dismay settling on the thousands still there. We had just about given up hope of hearing Tata Mandela speak. I was sitting on the ground in a sun-struck daze, with my head in my hands, when there was a roar of euphoria. The drifting currents of the crowd poured back into the vortex. Mandela had arrived at last. The distinctive timbre of his voice flowed over us as the summer sky dissolved into darkness.

It was both the most wonderful and the most dreadful day of my young life.

~ ~ ~

The ray of memory refracts through a prism, separating the momentous from the mundane. As if it were yesterday, I feel the impact of that first glimpse of his face. How different he looked from the 1960s photographs, which were the last most of us had seen of him! Then the prism shifts, the light bends, and I can taste the nausea of the heat exhaustion that laid me low for days afterwards, probe the stinging blister that festered on my sunburnt lip.

I have had many privileges, and one of them was hearing the rising tide of Tata Mandela's voice washing over his tired people, weary from hours of waiting, weary from centuries of waiting. Within two minutes, he'd made a commitment to the South African nation to 'place the remaining years of my life in your hands'. This was a pledge behind which he stood until his death at the age of ninety-five. His final months were hard. I'm glad he is at rest now, after a lifetime of service to his country. His party may have disappointed many of us in the decades following his presidency, but he never did.

~ ~ ~

In the months that followed, while I never suffered anything close to the same hardships and dangers faced by my Black comrades, I did learn what it was to be afraid.

The bitter huddle over burning newspaper as we gasped through clouds of teargas.

The favourite T-shirt I pulled from my pack to bind the leg of a stranger, injured in a police baton charge. Her limb had been gashed through layers of skin and fat and muscle, and I woke from graphic nightmares of that weeping flesh for months.

The panic of falling, myself, in the stampede away from those same baton-wielding police. My boyfriend dragged me out from under hundreds of trampling feet but, like a Cinderella who'd danced at a particularly unenjoyable ball, all I lost was a single shoe. This was so often the aftermath of a police dispersal: a scattering of odd footwear strewn across the pavement. I didn't go home that night, so I had to attend university classes barefoot the next day. This sparked an argument. My boyfriend, who had grown up in a community of Black farm labourers where bare feet were shameful evidence of poverty, would have preferred me to borrow a pair of oversized men's clodhoppers.

And there was the summer morning when two men arrived at the bank where I worked in a low-level clerical job, greeting me with a snide 'Happy birthday for yesterday.' I had just turned nineteen. They claimed they were from 'Intelligence' but refused to provide identification. Then came the barrage of questions designed to intimidate, showing how much they already knew. This wasn't a big deal, considering the cruel power of the security police, but I knew well what others had suffered: the detentions, the disappearances, even the deaths.

I was a teenaged girl from the suburbs who had spent most of her life protected from the ugliness of what was going on in her own country, and I was sorely frightened. My safety net was significant but not invincible. Trade unionist Neil Aggett's white skin hadn't saved him from a noose in a police cell.

Like countless other South Africans who turned out for peaceful protests, I also endured the reeking furnace of a yellow lock-up truck parked in the sun. Grim police herded dozens of *toyi-toying* bodies inside, bolted the door with a clang, then left us to shake our metal jail with stamping feet, to sing out defiance as our sweat fouled the baking air.

Most of our demonstrations were marches, but sometimes we varied the program. The most dramatic protest I attended was a sit-in at the offices of the National Party, which had led the government for more than four decades. When their staff went home for the day, we refused to leave — at least until the police arrived and hauled us away. Somewhere, a lawyer later told me, there is footage of us laughing as we arranged an ANC flag like a turban around the bronze head of an apartheid ex-president's statue.

Far more restrained was the time I joined ranks with the Black Sash in one of their haunting stands, keeping silent watch on the steps of Nobel Peace Laureate Archbishop Desmond Tutu's cathedral.

The Black Sash was then an association of white women that had been campaigning against injustice since the 1950s.

They took real risks of police persecution and sometimes physical violence from hostile passersby. In his release speech, Nelson Mandela credited them — and the National Union of South African Students — for having acted 'as the conscience of white South Africans'. Anti-apartheid groups organised along racial lines made me uncomfortable, though, even if I grew to understand the reasons for their existence. It was Black Consciousness Movement icon Steve Biko who best explained that Black South Africans had to claim their own table, before they could invite white activists to sit at it.

~ ~ ~

By 1991, I had enrolled at the University of the Western Cape. UWC was a historically Black campus, a holdover from the not-so-distant times when the government restricted university admission by race. My parents were exasperated by my decision. They had raised me to take a moral stand against racism in my day-to-day life, but my political choices bewildered them. Plus, they were concerned I might be settling for an inferior education in an institution that had long been disadvantaged in government funding. Still, they supported me as they did all their children: paying my first year's tuition and standing surety for my bank loans for the next three years.

Finding a political home at UWC posed an unexpected problem. NUSAS, the progressive white students' organisation recognised by Mandela that day on the Grand Parade, wasn't an option. To the best of my knowledge, I was the only white full-time undergraduate for two of my four years at uni, and so, of course, there was no branch of NUSAS for me to join.

There was a branch of the South African National Students Congress, the body that had evolved from the organisation founded by Biko and other Black Consciousness activists when they broke away from NUSAS in the late 1960s. It took months, though, before I was allowed in. After all, SANSCO had been formed, in part, as a remedy against Black students being sidelined by (sometimes well-meaning) white activists. Its very constitution began with the preamble: 'Whereas we the Black students of South Africa, realising that we are members of an oppressed community before we are students…'

When, after closed deliberations, SANSCO welcomed me in, I was mindful of this history. In contrast to the rest of my political life, I kept my voice low, my presence unobtrusive, even after the two organisations re-merged in September 1991. I was grateful for the concession, although it took decades before the Black Lives Matter movement helped me appreciate its magnitude.

~ ~ ~

The world had applauded Mandela's release but, fifteen tumultuous months later, hundreds of activists were still behind bars and desperate not to be forgotten. Eighteen inmates on Robben Island — the maximum-security prison just off the coast of Cape Town where Mandela spent eighteen years of his sentence — announced a hunger strike.

Masses of people marched on Cape Town's parliament in solidarity. Community leaders tagged a few of us to run ahead and chain ourselves to the metal fence. We were only minutes from our objective, so there was no chance to confer or strategise. They simply handed us chains with open padlocks — no keys, as these would have made it too easy to remove our restraints — and we peeled away from our friends to lock ourselves down before police guarding the building caught wind of our plan.

Picture the scene: a pack of demonstrators chanting and swaying along Adderley Street, Cape Town's main drag. Adderley leads to Government Avenue, a tree-lined esplanade running between parliament and the pleasant park known as the Company's Garden. Seventeenth-century Dutch settlers planted this garden to grow vegetables for trading ships rounding the Cape of Good Hope on the long, scurvy-ridden voyage from Europe to the spice markets of Asia. The Dutch East India Company was as vicious a body of marauding predators as you could never hope to meet. Their garden, by contrast, is a tranquil botanical retreat, popular with workers on their lunch breaks, harbouring colonies of grey squirrels and a cluster of the city's museums. It is a frequent destination for school excursions.

I dashed ahead of the crowd and a short stretch up Government Avenue, wound the chain around my waist and through the fence rails, and snapped the heavy padlock shut with a triumphant *clunk*. As I leaned back, catching my breath, the march slowly approached, and slowly turned, and slowly made its way out of sight to the far side of the parliament buildings.

And there I stood.

Alone.

Except for two police officers sniggering in the landscaped grounds behind me.

An eternity passed in the fine red mist of humiliation. *What on earth am I going to do?* A gaggle of primary school kids trundled past two-by-two, following their teacher to a museum at the end of the now peaceful avenue. The teacher ignored me, but the children? They pointed and stared.

It was not my proudest moment. I don't recall who alerted the march leaders to my absence, but I do remember my relief when one of them trotted around the corner to unlock my chains. I got off lightly that time.

I didn't always get off so lightly, and, on four occasions, I was arrested. Once, there were only eight of us detained. After the police separated us by race and gender, I waited several anxious hours alone in a dim holding cell, the only white female in the group. Other times, I was one of scores, even hundreds, of demonstrators arrested, booked, then released, and the process was not as scary. While we were boisterous and undoubtedly troublesome, I was never involved in acts of violence.

All four of my arrests took place in 1990 and 1991, when we were campaigning to liberate political prisoners. Each arrest meant numerous days I had to take off work as we waited at the Cape Town Magistrate's Court for hours to learn whether our cases would be heard or, yet again, deferred. The first time, before we understood that this was a lengthy game being played, my mum came along to support me. She ended up making a grocery run to get sliced bread and sandwich ingredients, and handing them around to dozens of committed insurgents, my co-accused, waiting outside the courthouse.

In two cases, the authorities dropped the charges against us. In the others, there were preliminary date-setting hearings, but the cases never went to trial. Instead, pro-bono lawyers offered us the opportunity to pay admission-of-guilt fines of fifty Rand each. Today, this translates to about five Australian dollars, but it was more than twenty percent of my weekly pay. I never served any prison time.

Even after the delayed release of political prisoners, negotiations for the transition to democracy were far from smooth, and we continued our protests until the announcement that South Africa's first democratic election would be held on 27 April 1994.

As for me, activism was central to my identity for five years, from before my eighteenth birthday in 1989 until after South Africa's historic 1994 election. It was only when the revolutionary struggle evolved into party politics — followed by my move away from my community networks to work in a museum in Pretoria, 1,500 kilometres away — that my involvement diminished.

My beliefs haven't changed, as life has knocked me around over the decades, but my energy has bled away. I've become a person who hides from the news, overwhelmed by the injustice and suffering I see whenever I look up from my books. I should be doing more.

~ ~ ~

And what does all this have to do with my return to Greece?

I could never have guessed, all those years ago, that I would one day live across the world in Australia. Or that my nephew, who was just five years old when Nelson Mandela raised his fist as a free man, would grow up to work in Canada. Or that events from decades ago and a continent away might thwart my plans to visit him, and take me to Greece instead.

CHAPTER TWO
ON MY WAY TO CANADA...
OR NOT?

NOT HAVING CHILDREN OF my own, my nephews and nieces mean the world to me, even though they live worlds away. The desire to see my far-away family and my passion for exploring new lands often pull me in opposite directions but, this time, I'd be able to satisfy both urges at once. My nephew's company was sending him to Canada — a country I'd never visited — for months at a stretch. A meet-up with Christopher in Vancouver had been on my radar ever since he rented an apartment there in 2016.

Then his sister Carly took a sea change from her often-traumatic job riding the ambulances in Cape Town. She joined the medical team aboard a cruise ship that would pass, from time to time, through Vancouver on its way to Alaska. Seeing the two of them at once, anywhere but on a visit back home, would be a novelty. Plus, I'd get to know Karen, the woman Christopher loves. I had visions of a luxury train ride through

the Rockies with my nephew, shipboard cocktails with my
niece under a sky ablaze with surreal green flame, maybe
even a leisurely meal with the four of us sipping red wine
around Christopher's table, if Carly could get shore leave.

But trying to coordinate dates proved tricky, an unshared
cabin on Carly's ship cost more than I could afford, and I put
those dreams on hold when Greece so irresistibly drew me
to her shores in September 2016.

By early 2017, though, the radar's ping became more
insistent. I was saving up both dollars and leave days, and I
longed to see Christopher and meet Karen. I'd adjusted my
expectations — there'd be a budget bus to Banff, rather than
the opulent train called the Rocky Mountaineer — and I was
eager to set foot in Canada.

My niece, a true nomad, had moved on to sail other seas.
That was an opportunity missed. *But,* I told myself, *at least
scheduling will be easier. And there'll always be other opportunities
to see Carly.*

After Christopher and I settled on May for the visit, I
looked into travel requirements and was once again struck by
how privileged I was to hold dual citizenship: entry to so many
countries had become a breeze. Australian passport-holders
didn't even need a visa to enter Canada. All we needed was
something called an eTA, or Electronic Travel Authorization,
which, the official website explained, would typically be
granted a few seconds after filling out the online application.

Organising an international trip can be a juggle as there are so many factors affecting your flight dates. It's unwise to buy a plane ticket before your boss approves your leave, but the dates of travel may depend on fluctuating airfares. You can't purchase insurance until the dates are set, but it's best to get immediate coverage in case something forces you to cancel your getaway. Technically, you shouldn't commit to travel without a visa or, in this case, an eTA. But a visa application might ask for specific dates or even flight numbers... which are contingent on approved leave... which will depend on daily ticket prices... and so it goes. The arrangements can get in such a tangle that it's hard for even an experienced traveller to know where to start.

At last, the juggling was done. Dates were set, leave approved, air tickets printed, insurance cover secured. The only task left was to apply for the eTA.

This is where it all began to go pear-shaped.

~ ~ ~

In February 2017, as I sat down to my computer in small-town Australia to apply for a Canadian eTA, I was blissfully unaware that I was about to be swamped in a morass of bureaucracy.

It was a simple form and I sped through it, ticking the boxes. My first misgivings came when I got to the question, 'Have you ever committed, been arrested for, been charged with or convicted of any criminal offence in any country/territory?'

Honest to a fault, I ticked yes.

After supplying a brief explanation in the limited characters permitted, I clicked on the submission button. Instead of the instantaneous approval I'd been expecting, an ominous email appeared in my inbox. It asked for a plethora of documents before a human would look at my application.

> Police Certificate: Please provide an original police clearance certificate An Australian National Police Certificate — Standard Disclosure — name check ISSUED EXCLUSIVELY by the Australian Federal Police, issued within 6 months from the date you submitted your application. Please note: a police certificate issued by a state authority is NOT ACCEPTABLE. This must be received at this office by: 2017/03/24

> Court record / Police report: Please provide the court dispositions for the offence(s) mentioned on your application form. The court dispositions must state the section(s) of the law under which you were convicted. Please note, if you were convicted of an offence involving alcohol, the court dispositions must state the section of the

law under which you were convicted as well as your blood or breath alcohol level at the time of the offence. This must be received at this office by: 2017/03/24

Police Certificate: Please provide an original police clearance certificate from South Africa. The Police Certificate must be issued within six months from the date of your application. This must be received at this office by: 2017/03/24

Before I'd finished working through the bureaucratic language, I'd reached for my antacids. Eyes on the screen, my thumbs pressed a tablet from its blister pack. I wasn't too concerned about the Canadian authorities deeming me unfit to enter their country. I've always been honest when asked about my arrest record and, without exception, people have been reasonable once I've had a chance to explain. But this was going to be a major hassle. And a pricey one.

The Aussie certificate cost forty-two dollars and it was a mystery why the Canadians wanted it, given that the arrests happened a decade and a half before my Australian immigration, but the application was painless, and the document arrived within a few weeks.

I wasn't going to be able to produce any court records or police reports related to the arrests, but I was optimistic that, once I could account for why these weren't available, all would be well.

The third requirement would be the biggest hurdle. I already had three South African police clearance certificates, dated 1998, 2000 and 2007, but to get a current one from across the world would be expensive and time-consuming. There wasn't a day to waste, so I stopped by my local police station first thing next morning.

They had taken my prints at this station when I renewed my South African passport a few years earlier. It had been a simple matter. I had popped in before work with a fingerprint form supplied by the South African High Commission, and a helpful police officer had rolled my fingers in ink at the front counter amid laughing banter from his colleagues.

This time, the man at the front desk informed me that they no longer processed fingerprints there, and that I would have to phone to schedule a time at another police station, a train ride away. I managed to get an appointment for the following day, and Adam — my partner of nine years — saved me the commute by giving me a lift and waiting outside for me to get inked.

A police officer in her early twenties ushered me into the holding area and lined me up at the digital fingerprint machine. Recalling strict instructions from the South African consulate when I had my passport renewed, I explained I might need to provide ink fingerprints.

She seemed doubtful. 'That's not how we do it these days. It's all electronic.'

'Nevertheless,' I persisted.

A shelf in the corner near the holding cell doors held tired fingerprint forms, all labelled 'MALE'. With a slight air of humouring an old fogey, the officer scrabbled around in drawers until she located an inkpad and forms for females. We chatted about my upcoming Canadian trip as she inked my fingers and palms, then pressed and rolled them on the paper.

Our heads together, we examined the end product. My smudged prints were no clearer than a child's finger painting. She offered to make a digital set at no extra charge, an offer I accepted with gratitude. While swiping my credit card to pay the fee, I asked the civilian office staff if they could stamp the printed forms with an official stamp, but they turned me down with a dismissive, 'We don't do that.'

At home, we scrutinised the quality of the two sets of prints. Adam, a firefighter, would be attending a training course with other emergency services personnel the next day, and he decided to show the inked form to a senior police officer. She agreed the prints were useless. I would have to send in the digital set.

While I chased the ink, Megan, my closest friend since high school, was looking into the South African side of things. With every day crucial, she recommended a company that facilitated police checks for employers vetting job candidates.

For a fee, this company would submit the application. They'd then stop by the South African Criminal Records Centre three times a week to check whether the certificate was ready for collection. There was one hitch: they advised Megan the fingerprint form must bear a police station date stamp. I'd have to call the Australian police and plead my case.

To my bewilderment, the cheerful lady who answered the phone said that *of course* they could stamp the digital printout, no problem at all. Off we went to get it stamped.

I had now compiled my application pack to send to South Africa. It included a cover letter, the Canadian request, copies of the three out-of-date police clearance certificates, the digital fingerprint form (duly stamped), copies of my South African identity document and passport, and proof of payment of both the police fee and the bill for the company following up on the application. I scanned the fat sheaf of documents and emailed it to Megan to have the company check that all was in order before I committed this important package to the post.

It wasn't. Digital prints were not acceptable. And, despite the information on the South African Police Service website that fingerprints of citizens living outside the Republic 'should be taken on the official fingerprint forms of the specific country', they strongly advised me to provide the prints on a South African form 91(a), which Megan was able to send via email. The police website made no mention of ink, or date stamps for that matter, but I didn't want to take any chances.

In the car, a long-suffering Adam wondered aloud why, if he kept taking me to the police station, they kept on letting me go.

This time, a police officer of about my age lost no time in pulling out the real fingerprint ink. She gave a slow shake of her head when I told her about the regular office inkpad the friendly young officer had used before. This was the good stuff: sticky black ink trapped between sheets of plastic. When she peeled them apart, they provided the perfect surface for coating every ridge and whorl. The latest version of the fingerprint form was a work of art. A quick date stamp, and I was on my way.

By then, stressful weeks had passed, and the documents had yet to leave Australia's shores.

The package took six days to get to South Africa, and another five to reach the vetting company making the application on my behalf. Then the waiting game started. The police website quoted a turnaround time of fourteen days. The company said it was more likely to be four to six weeks. Some online browsing scared me with stories it could take up to six months. Meanwhile, the deadline from the Canadians, 24 March, was fast approaching. There was an online portal to submit the documents, so I sat at my computer and did what I could.

I uploaded the Australian Federal Police certificate, crossing one requirement off the list.

At the request for court documents, I submitted a grovelling plea. I explained that, when I'd applied for permanent residency in Australia, I'd spent ages trying to track down official records, ending up at the National Archives of South Africa. There, a patient attendant told me that Magistrates' Court documentation from the 1990s had not been digitised or even thoroughly sorted. The files were stored in cardboard boxes, many of them damaged by damp. He helped me search through those cartons he was able to locate, but we couldn't find any court dispositions.

As for the South African police certificate: I supplied the three old certificates, and proof I had applied for a new one. I also detailed the nature of the arrests and expressed my concern that a current document wouldn't arrive in time for the trip.

Surely, now I've had an opportunity to clarify what happened, the Canadians will let me in?

They didn't. Still, they dropped their request for court documentation — a huge relief — and extended the deadline for the police certificate until 19 April.

Now all I had to do was wait. And worry. About the timeframe, but also about another potential problem I'd been trying to push from my mind. It had grown from fretful anxiety to choking dread. Because even if the certificate arrived on time, I didn't know what it would say.

Technically, it should show two of my four arrests, the ones where I had paid the admission-of-guilt fines to avoid lengthy court cases. But the first two times I applied for certificates, in 1998 and 2000, they stated that I had no convictions recorded against me. I assumed the records for minor anti-apartheid infringements had been expunged. But the certificate issued in 2007, when I was collating documents for my Australian residential visa application, nearly blew up my immigration plans.

It recorded in aggressive all caps that, in October 1990, I had been convicted of 'DISPLAYING A FIRE-ARM AT A PUBLIC GATHERING'.

This was the reason I had tried so hard to find court records in the run-up to my move to Australia. Claiming, 'I've never touched a gun in my life!' would count for nothing. Luckily, a reasonable official shared my interpretation of the only document I could find — a handwritten record, in scrawled Afrikaans, from the old police station case book. It showed I was number 34 in a long list of demonstrators arrested together — hardly the case if I had been brandishing a weapon. There was no way members of a large group of armed insurgents would get to walk away with no trial and a fifty Rand fine. In a victory for common sense, the certificate was reissued with the conviction shown as 'ATTENDING AN ILLEGAL GATHERING OR DEMONSTRATION'.

But now? Who knew what message my 2017 document might carry?

Anxious weeks followed. Every morning I awoke with the hope that the South Africans had emailed the certificate during the Australian night, and every morning my heart sank a little lower. The day before the April deadline, I submitted an even more eloquent appeal for the authorities to approve my application based on the information I'd already provided. When I received their response, my spirit broke. Not only were they insisting on a current police certificate, but they had revived their demand for court documents, the very records I had explained possibly didn't exist and certainly weren't available. They did grant another extension, though: until 19 May, six days before my booked flight to Vancouver.

At last, I awoke one Saturday morning to the email from South Africa I had so desperately been awaiting. The attached police certificate showed one conviction, described in vague terms as 'PROHIBITION OF CERTAIN GATHERING AND DEMONSTRATIONS IN THE DEFINED AREA'.

A weight rolled off my shoulders. The drama of obtaining this certificate had cost more than $160 in Aussie dollars, a lot of sleepless nights and a few grey hairs. I uploaded the police certificate and explained once again why I couldn't produce court documents. There was nothing more I could do. *At least now I'll get an answer*, I thought, *and soon*. I'd received responses to the previous three submissions within hours, sometimes minutes. With more than three weeks until my departure date, I felt a glimmer of optimism.

It took four days to receive an acknowledgement email from an address marked 'DoNotReply'. A week later, I called my nephew and warned him our get-together was beginning to seem unlikely. Referring to a catchphrase from our favourite author, Terry Pratchett, Christopher intoned the magic words, 'It's a million-to-one chance, but it might just work.' He shushed me when I claimed it wasn't yet quite as dire as that. The odds must be *exactly* a million to one, he reminded me, for it to turn out okay.

With under a fortnight until my flight date, I had to come up with a Plan B. After half a year in a job that didn't suit my skills or interests, I had won a secondment to an exciting new position, due to start on my first day back from leave. If I didn't get the Canadian approval, I could scrap my holiday, accept the monetary loss — my insurance wouldn't cover this one — and go straight to the new role. But that would be too depressing for words. The last few months had been horrible, workwise. Even my writing had stalled, a couple of chapters shy of completing my first travel memoir. I needed a rejuvenating break, and to use the time simply to hang out at home would be such a waste.

Then came a flash of inspiration: *Eureka! If I can't go to Canada, I'll return to Greece. I'll take Mum's diary back to the islands she walked, four decades ago. And I'll find the ending of my book.* I looked up Greek flights, and the best option would leave Sydney on the evening of 24 May, ten hours earlier than my proposed flight to Vancouver.

On 18 May, I had a serious discussion with my nephew. My attempt to contact the Canadians through their webform had led to an automatic response saying the turnaround time for a reply would be ten business days, almost a week *after* I was supposed to board the plane. The deadline for receiving a partial refund on the tickets was 22 May. I wasn't comfortable waiting until the last minute, not least because that was the date my travel agent Chantel, who knew the backstory and would be processing the cancellation, was due to give birth to her second child. Plus, a trip to Greece would require more organising than I could manage in two days, both of which would be busy workdays at that.

Christopher and I agreed that the cut-off for changing my plans would be lunchtime on Friday 19 May in Australia, aligning with close of business on Thursday afternoon, Canadian time.

It was a million-to-one chance. It didn't work.

Lunchtime came and went. I broke the news to Christopher via Facebook Messenger and contacted Chantel, who did a sterling job of cancelling one set of tickets and purchasing another between contractions (mild ones, she assured me).

At 1.35 p.m. on Monday 22 May, I received an email from the Canadian immigration service, stating, 'Please be advised that your eTA application has been approved.'

It was too late. It had been a busy weekend. I'd cancelled my tickets to Vancouver at a cost of $480, booked and paid for tickets to Greece and three internal flights, reserved accommodation. I had made new plans, and it would be unreasonable to change them again. The timing of the approval was devastating, although there was some consolation in the eTA granting a five-year window in which I could visit my nephew.

And that's how I came to make an unexpected landing at Athens Eleftherios Venizelos International Airport, just eight months after my first visit to Greece.

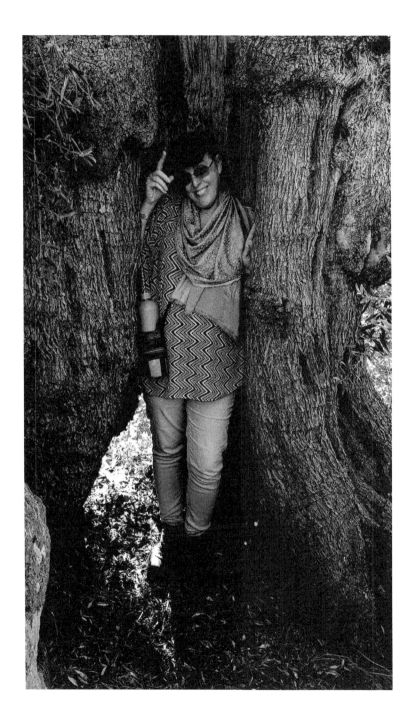

FINDING PEACE:
A GENTLER ODYSSEY

CHAPTER THREE
ATHENS AGAIN

I couldn't go to Canada, so I flew back to Greece, with my mother's 1978 travel journal once again tucked into my pocket.

And, oh, how different it was coming into Athens this time around. Instead of a daunting series of obstacles, the ride from the airport was a comfortable commute. Last year, I'd had to find the metro, buy a ticket in an unknown language with unfamiliar currency, work out the connections, and worry about finding my way from train station to hotel. This time, rather than sitting at the edge of my seat to peer out the window at every station signboard, I settled back, thankful to be on the final leg of a long journey.

I even remembered a few phrases from the last trip. Jumping right into it, I excused myself with a polite '*Sygnómi*' as I gestured for a man to step aside so I could get my snazzy new suitcase off the luggage rack. Then I thanked him like a pro with an '*Efcharistó*' and smiled at his '*Parakaló*'. My smug grin faded when he went back to talking with his buddies in German. We'd both been practicing our tourist Greek.

I was staying at the family-run Art Gallery Hotel again, so I knew where to go and how to get there. It was like coming home to a friend's house, with an amiable greeting from a familiar face as I walked in the door. All that was missing was Arti, the hotel's tuxedo cat, who had ventured out to roam the neighbourhood before I arrived.

He could keep his nocturnal escapades. I was happy with a quiet night, and it wasn't long before I was fast asleep.

~ ~ ~

At sunrise, I woke to discover that the previous night's mild headache — caused by a careless passenger pulling his luggage from the plane's overhead compartment and clipping my head with his suitcase wheels — had become a splitting one. That wasn't the only mishap of the flight. The pretty flamenco fan I'd bought four years earlier, when I visited Barcelona with my friend Megan, had splintered at some point during the last thirty-six hours. And now, when I tried to close the zipper of the foldaway daypack she'd given me as we parted in Venice, it jammed halfway.

Yesterday's high had dimmed. Today's long-distance bus ride was looming and an old anxiety had risen with the sun. I'd thought my first journey through Greece had conquered the fear of road travel that had dogged my steps since one bus crashed into another in rural Sri Lanka, leaving me broken. *Turns out I was wrong*, I thought, frustrated at how difficult it was to shake off the past.

The night in an unfamiliar bed had left me with a dull ache in my left shoulder, recalling my old injury. I dropped the fan in the bin with regret and the pack on my bed to deal with later, shoved the rest of my belongings back into my bags and dosed my head with painkillers. My bus to Delphi wouldn't leave until 3.00 pm, so I started out for a stroll in the cool morning air.

Ten minutes on foot took me to the rocky hill of the Acropolis. I skirted the carpark and made for the Pnyx, the grassy field where Athenians once gathered to vote in the city's earliest democratic assemblies. Then, taking a wrong turn, I stumbled upon the overgrown stone paving of the Koile road that Dimitri, the charismatic guide who had so infected me with his enthusiasm last year, had mentioned. He wasn't the only one; Herodotus, who may have been the world's first historian, wrote about this thoroughfare two and a half thousand years ago. As I walked through the scrubby vegetation at the side of the ancient road, I inhaled the earthy aromas set free by the May morning's brief downpour. Each step I took heightened my awareness of once again grounding myself in Greece. With every breath came a gradual release of the iron clamp gripping my temples.

Heading back towards the Acropolis, I turned up a track that passed three grille-covered caves signposted as 'the "Prison of Socrates"', the tentative punctuation signalling that archaeologists no longer believed this to be where the troublesome philosopher spent the night before his death. Socrates may or may not have visited these ancient caves, but I knew from my mother's diary that she had trodden this same trail in 1978. I rested my hand on the scarred rockface and wondered whether she might have pressed her fingers into this same stone.

At the church of Saint Dimitrios Loumbardiaris I found — how splendid! — that today its doors stood open, unlike both times I'd tried them during my first trip.

The church's chancel was a cave-like sanctuary of brick and plaster. The icon displayed in pride of place portrayed a green-cloaked saint who must have been Dimitrios. In its lower right corner, the icon showed the Acropolis beneath his horse's rearing hooves and, under the point of the saint's great spear, the cannon with which Yusuf the Turk menaced the church. Bunches of ribbon-tied *tamata* dangled from the icon's heavy wooden frame. These tin-thin rectangles, embossed with images, were symbolic of prayers to the saint. As I gazed at miniature depictions of a man, an arm, a woman, and a pair of eyes, I wondered what ailments they represented and added my good wishes to the petitioners' appeals.

A lady dressed in widow's black, although she couldn't have been much older than me, confirmed that this was indeed the icon of Saint Dimitrios. When she invited me to take a candle, I slipped a euro into the collection box and told her this would be for *mitéra mou*. Using gestures more fluent than her few words of English, she asked why I was lighting a candle for my mother. When I told her Mum had died, her smile turned sorrowful and she wished me *kooráyio*, courage.

It was beyond my ability to explain that my mum had been dead for almost twenty years and the grief was not new, but that I wanted to honour her here because she would have seen this church. She would have passed it on her path to the caves known as the prison of Socrates.

My 2016 itinerary had been booked before my sisters reminded me about Mum's visit to Greece, before I even knew her travel diary existed. Last year, those caves had been my first Greek touchpoint with my mother, but my way had soon diverged from hers. This time was different: I had chosen to come back to Greece precisely so I could tread in her footsteps, using her journal to plot my path. She hadn't seen much of the country — she'd only been here for three nights — but she had visited the Saronic islands of Aegina, Poros and Hydra. It was fitting that my trip would culminate in the Saronic Gulf, and that it started with this little church.

By now, it was nearing eleven o'clock, and I returned to tourism central in the hope of achieving my mission for the morning: to locate Dimitri, the tour guide who had opened my heart to the marvels of Greece during my first trip to Athens. I wanted to thank him, and to pay him the courtesy of letting him know about the book I was writing. Disappointingly, he wasn't working that day. One of his colleagues flipped open her satchel and extracted a notebook with an image of Al-Khazneh, the most-renowned monument of Petra in Jordan's desert, on its cover. She ripped out a page so I could leave Dimitri a message.

I wasn't prepared for this. The news of my book was far too complex and personal to share in a brief note composed on the spur of a jet-lagged moment, but I jotted a few lines, taking care to include my email address in my neatest handwriting:

Dimitri,

I was on your walking tour last September and it was a wonderful introduction to Athens and Greece. There is something I would like to tell you. Please could you email me?

Efcharistó
Sally

It's possible I was too cryptic, because Dimitri never contacted me. Maybe he didn't receive the note. Or thought I was some creepy stalker type. Perhaps he meant to reply but never got around to it.

~ ~ ~

This fleeting contact with Dimitri's colleague bore a significance disproportionate to the casual generosity with which she offered that scrap of paper. The randomness of the notebook's appearance, at a time when my mother's presence was strong in my mind, sparked a momentary shock of memory.

A framed postcard of the rose-red Nabatean city of Petra has hung on my bedroom walls on three continents, so far. It is a place my mother yearned to visit but never had the chance. It was on her bucket list long before any of us had heard that catchphrase.

The effect of pop culture on this ancient site mirrors what happened at Greece's Meteora, where a James Bond movie altered the economic and cultural landscape, causing many monks to flee to the religious enclave of Mount Athos. In a similar tale of unintended consequences, Steven Spielberg directed parts of *Indiana Jones and the Last Crusade* at Petra in the late 1980s, leading to an explosion in visitor numbers and concern for the damage that less-than-responsible tourism is causing at this World Heritage Site.

I made my own pilgrimage to Jordan in south-west Asia to see Petra a few years after my mother's death. Access to the site is by foot through a narrow canyon, the Siq, which twists for more than a kilometre between natural rock walls that rise up to 182 metres on either side. As we approached the end of the gorge, our guide told me to close my eyes. He took my hand, his rough palm hot against mine, and led me forward a few steps before whispering to me to open them.

It was as if a glowing beam had ruptured dark clouds. Instead of the forbidding red walls hemming us in, the majestic mausoleum of Al-Khazneh shimmered, gilded in sunlight, in the air before us. A powerful sensation engulfed me: *I'm here because my mother can't be.*

I also have a less poetic memory of my mother's fascination with Petra. Back in the 1990s, she owned a desktop computer but refused to use it for anything other than playing Solitaire. After we lost my dad to an unexpected heart attack, and a variety of events led to four of her six children living overseas, we convinced her to try email. The results were an eccentric joy to read. She hadn't mastered the art of the Enter key, so she used the spacebar to move to a new line, not understanding that each computer's settings would interpret her quirky formatting differently. Her staggered sentences danced all over my screen. At Christmas, she used a clumsy Paint program to draw a picture of the nativity, a waving foot the sole visible sign of Jesus in his manger.

Living alone for the first time in her life, my mother was bored. She had been ill for years, suffering from the debilitating disease called scleroderma that would kill her in the end, and this limited her ability to take up new interests. It was hard to help from Chile, where I'd moved to be with a man I'd met in an online chatroom, but I tried to get her to delve into the World Wide Web. The internet had changed my life; I hoped it would enhance hers.

When I succeeded in my persuasions, it was to dire effect.

Giving her the address of a pre-Google search engine, I urged, 'Mum, you can find out so much about any subject under the sun. Think about somewhere you would like to explore. How about Petra? You've always said how much you'd love to go there. Type in "Petra" and see what happens.'

Who could have guessed the first link would be to 'Petra's Palace of Pleasure'? My poor mother, a religious and socially conservative woman, landed in a hardcore porn site. To make matters worse, the webpage opened endless pop-ups each time she tried to close the window. As far as I know, my mum never used a search engine again.

~ ~ ~

In the foyer of the Art Gallery Hotel, I found a feline in disgrace. My Facebook friends got to know Arti during my first visit to Greece, and I knew they'd want an update:

26 May 2017

Arti the hotel cat is back, and disdainfully ignoring
the hotelier, who said they had to use a ladder to
retrieve him from a balcony in the neighbouring
apartment block. 'And it's not the first time,' she
remarked caustically.

With a haughty flick of his tail, Arti turned his back and
lay down for a nap. Considering this a dismissal, I collected
my luggage from a utility room behind the reception area and
refilled my bottle with tepid tap water at a little sink. I fitted
the bottle into the colourful Peruvian sling I'd been carrying
around the world since my sisters, niece and I attempted
the Inca Trail in 2001, then towed my suitcase out into busy
Athens in search of a bus to board. I was on my way to Delphi
to visit the navel of the Earth and walk the paths of the oracle.

CHAPTER FOUR
ATHENS TO DELPHI, AND A SIDE TRIP

I N PERU, THE OLD Inca capital city of Cuzco takes its name from the indigenous Quechuan word *qosq'o*, meaning 'the navel of the Earth'. But it appears our planet has more than one belly button. Zeus, leader of the Greek gods, pinpointed the centre of the world by setting two eagles in flight from opposite ends of the Earth. He cast down a boulder to mark the spot where their flight paths crossed, declaring it the navel of the Earth. This stone, the Omphalos, sits amid the glory of Delphi, on the slopes of magnificent Mount Parnassus.

When I'd announced on social media that I might return to Greece to seek the end of a story I was writing, my sister Jenny was quick to respond. I hadn't yet told her how a chance Peruvian recollection during my first Greek trip, together with a handwritten date in our mother's diary, had caused a sudden shift in my relationship with Mum's memory. Nevertheless, knowing the manuscript had become something of a tribute to our mum, she commented, 'You'll need to finish at Mount Parnassus. When the world was destroyed, that's where it got to start again. Funny thing is that it starts with the bones of their mother.'

I'd never heard of Mount Parnassus or its role in the rebirth of humanity, but it wasn't hard to find the story. It was a familiar tale, echoing other flood myths from around the world: from Hinduism, to Norse mythology, to the story of Noah and his ark that my mother used to teach to children from our church. Her catechism classes took place in our hideously wallpapered dining room when I was about four years old, with my mother instructing the neighbourhood kids using paper cut-outs of Biblical characters stuck onto a fuzzy felt backdrop. Those cut-out characters served a dual purpose: a teaching aid for the older students, and a bribe for me — if I behaved impeccably, I'd be allowed to play out my own felt-and-paper stories after the class.

There are a few variations of the Greek legend of Mount Parnassus but, in essence, it tells how Deucalion (son of Prometheus, who stole fire from the gods and gifted it to humankind) and his wife Pyrrha (daughter of Pandora, who let out the evils of the world) escaped a deluge sent by Zeus.

Prometheus warned his son that Zeus was planning to wipe out human civilisation in a terrible flood. Deucalion built a great chest in which the couple floated for nine days before it grounded in the Parnassus mountains. There, an oracle told them they could repopulate the Earth by tossing the bones of their mother behind them. They understood this to mean that they should cast the stones of Mother Earth over their shoulders. The rocks thrown by Deucalion changed into men, while those thrown by Pyrrha became women.

And so my itinerary was built, from Delphi nestled in the foothills of Mount Parnassus — which my mother hadn't visited — to the Saronic islands — which she had — and a few other wonders of Greece in between. Rhodes was conspicuous in its absence from the list. That temptation was too fresh to risk again.

I brought Mum's diary with me, but I was no longer trying to force a connection with her. I'd come to terms with it: my mother and I had little in common. If we had met as two adult women, it's unlikely we would have 'clicked' as friends. That's okay, though. It used to hurt more, to admit I lacked a sense of belonging with her. But it was enough, for now, to have caught a glimpse of who she was when she wasn't being my mum. In a weird way, this unfamiliar version of her, stored between scuffed covers, had become my travel companion, and had brought me peace.

~ ~ ~

Getting to Liosion Bus Terminal proved a bit tricky, involving a metro and a bus that set me down at the edge of a busy street, with the driver gesturing which way to walk to the terminus. I arrived in good time, though, and was soon sitting on the coach speeding north to Delphi.

First, we had to drive through miles and miles of gritty Athens.

Athens is a city of such odd contrasts. State-of-the-art infrastructure sits alongside charming, cobbled lanes cluttered with outdoor cafés. Today's dishevelled grunge surrounds oases of ancient elegance. As Dimitri had quipped during his tour the previous year, turning from the gracious monuments of old to a sprawl of lacklustre apartment blocks stretching to the horizon, 'I hope you like what we've done with the place.'

The skies were beautiful, though, with pale light gleaming through brooding clouds, their darkness fringed with fluffy white and slashed with whorls of vivid blue. Before the storm hit, we motored past a matte-black stone church, built in an otherwise Byzantine style, rubbing shoulders with the grubby buildings along the highway. Even the exit ramps seemed dramatic, their signs yelling '*EXODUS*' in booming Greek capital letters.

Then we entered a bright cloud of mist. Raindrops wriggled their diagonal way down the windowpanes, thunder crashed, and white light streamed through the windscreen. The shabbily genteel man in the seat next to me nodded off, unable to resist the pull of sleep.

There was something hypnotic about the smooth drone of the engine as we glided through the eerie glow, and it wasn't until the storm cleared that I remembered I was supposed to be afraid of bus travel. We were driving between farmland on our right and craggy hills on our left, both interrupted by occasional pockets of ugly industry. As we turned off near Thiva, the landscape transformed into a plateau of green and gold. Six human figures were bending and dipping along the furrows in a field.

Amid the patchwork of more conventionally coloured countryside were grey-blue squares of low-lying solar panels. This was a modern crop I would see sprouting throughout this Grecian journey, along with great wind turbines stalking across the ridges of the mainland like benevolent giants.

The bus slowed to a crawl. Far ahead, three men balanced precariously on a tractor pulling a ramshackle cart, their slow progress holding up a long line behind them. Even before I saw the driver's Sikh turban, they reminded me of the eccentric array of vehicles Adam and I had observed in India during a recent yoga tour, and the suppressed panic I felt every time we'd taken to the chaotic roads. I flashed the tractor's passengers a smile as we overtook, recalling the great works of Sikh charity we'd witnessed in the kitchens of the Golden Temple in Amritsar. *If I hadn't had to confront the snarling traffic in India, with Adam by my side to give me courage,* I wondered, *would I ever have dared set out alone for Greece?*

By the time I arrived at Pitho Rooms, where the owners' cheerful young son helped me lug my bags up the staircase, I was hungry for my first authentic Greek meal of the trip. At the restaurant across the road, windows reached from floor to ceiling and wall to wall. I'd come to Delphi for its World Heritage Site ruins, but no one had prepared me for the jaw-dropping grandeur of the terrain.

I posted the first of a series of Facebook photographs titled 'Delphi. The things you don't know until you get there.' It showed the folds of the hills sinking their feet into a soft plain that flowed all the way to the sea:

> 26 May 2017
> The majestic splendour of the landscape. This was just a small part of it, my view over a dinner of stuffed cabbage leaves in lemon sauce and deep-fried zucchini with tzatziki. A plateau carpeted with olive groves to the Gulf of Corinth.

I would have two nights in Delphi but only one full day, and there were a couple of places I hoped to visit in addition to the famed archaeological sites.

One of these was the village of Distomo, where Nazis slaughtered more than two hundred people in two hours of reprisals after a partisan ambush in 1944. The slain included the elderly in their eighties and babes in arms. Taking into account those murdered in the days after the massacre, the final death toll was 218.

This history evoked the Greece I'd read about in Nicholas Gage's *Eleni*, a harrowing memoir set during the Second World War and the brutal civil war that tore the country apart after the invaders left. It didn't feel right to come to this region without honouring the memory of those who'd died, and the suffering of the survivors left behind.

The other was a second World Heritage Site, one very different from the famous Delphi ruins, which I wouldn't have known was nearby if not for my *Lonely Planet* travel guide. About thirty-five kilometres away, on the slopes of Mount Helicon, lies Moni Osios Loukas. This monastery is dedicated to a local hermit, Saint Luke, who died in the year 953 CE and whose relics lie in state in a glass casket in the Katholikon. Its chapel, dating to the tenth century, may well be the oldest surviving church in mainland Greece.

That night, I pieced together information from my guidebook and the Athens-to-Delphi bus timetable I'd photographed at Liossion. Lying in my narrow bed, I concocted a convoluted plan for the limited time available.

I plotted each detail of the coming day. After a quick breakfast, I'd walk to the free archaeological sites outside the fenced Delphi complex. Then I would catch the eleven o'clock Athens bus and ask the driver to drop me at the turnoff to Distomo. My feet could take me the kilometre or so into town, where I would pay a taxi to transport me to the monastery and wait for me there. Back in Distomo, I would find a quiet place to remember the victims of the massacre. There'd be time for a meal before trekking to the main road and flagging down the next bus from Athens, which I estimated would come through sometime after 5.30 p.m. That should get me to Delphi just in time for a fleeting visit to the museum before it closed at eight o'clock. I would have to skip the hotel breakfast on my second morning to visit the major Delphi archaeological sites before catching the eleven o'clock bus to Athens.

It was complicated, and I would be exhausted, but I pushed away my apprehension that the bus driver wouldn't notice me waving at the side of the highway on my way back from Distomo. As I sank into sleep, I resolved it was doable.

The next morning, I woke even earlier than planned — a beneficial symptom of my jet lag. I crept downstairs and let myself out the hotel's locked front door long before breakfast. Already ahead of schedule, I made my way out of the town.

It was an easy walk under dawn-lit clouds, and the mountain air was sharp and fresh in the hours before the tourist coaches arrived from the city, dragging invisible contrails of diesel fumes behind them. Honeysuckle sweetened the breeze as I passed the path leading to the archaeological compound. Continuing along the road, I curved past the ancient gymnasium before coming to a spurt of clear water splashing from a spout into a stone trough. I cupped the liquid in my hand and sipped. The icy chill was a shock against my teeth.

Adjacent were the remains of the Castalian Spring where pilgrims once bathed to purify themselves before visiting the oracle. From the road, mossy steps descended to a paved courtyard flanked by a stone bench. A wire gate blocked a path climbing upwards, maybe to the spring itself. When I tugged at the locked gate, the rattle woke two dogs who lived in the rocky hills high above. They barked with joy, revelling in their guard duty, and I was happy to give them the pleasure of seeing me off their territory.

After passing a sign warning of rockfalls, I arrived above the jewel of Delphi, the Sanctuary of Athena Pronaia. Its name — meaning 'before' — has a double significance. It refers both to the foresight of the goddess and to her shrine's location as a gateway leading long-ago travellers to the temple quarter.

Three graceful pillars are all that remain of the circular *tholos* devoted to Athena. Together with the jagged stones standing in regular lines before them, they make up the best-known image of Delphi. This is not the place of the oracle, though. In fact, it lies well outside the present-day archaeological complex that encompasses the Temple of Apollo, where the prophetess communicated her visions to believers from many lands.

I was the first person to enter Athena's Sanctuary that morning.

Okay, instead of following that statement with something poetic about the morning light, I'll admit it: a gate blocked the path, stretching from a stone wall on one side to a steep drop-off on the other. A chain and padlock held it firmly closed. And time was short; if I left now, there'd be little chance of returning. Not without sacrificing another of the day's destinations, anyway.

Making an honest effort to identify any damage I might trigger through entering early, I ran through a mental checklist:

Financial harm? Zero. There was no admission fee.

Hazards to the archaeological remains? Zero. The site was designed for crowds of tourists, so a single person adhering to the walking trails should cause no negative impact.

Safety concerns? Zero. The only reason I could fathom for the gate's existence was to discourage lone wanderers who might injure themselves and lie undiscovered overnight. This danger did not apply, as the site would open within an hour. And the gate itself was a token barrier; it didn't pose any risk.

I wrestled with temptation and lost. Grabbing the top of the gate, I swung myself around its edge, over the stream that bubbled with youthful zest where the ground fell away abruptly at the side of the path. The energy of the cascading water was contagious, and I caught myself feeling a little bit younger.

Following a second gushing brook, I strode down to the temples and treasuries of old. At ground level, the tooth-like blocks of stone — so striking in photographs taken from above — were less pronounced, their surprising height and the surrounding vegetation hiding the serried ranks behind. Rushing water sang its song all around, and the rough-textured trunks of gnarled olive trees were a strangely soothing balm to the eyes. The solitude calmed me, and, as I climbed back up to the now-open gate, I relinquished my cumbersome scheme for the day. This would be the last time I'd fall into the trap of allowing unnecessary anxiety to govern my holiday plans. Instead of tying my arrangements into a tangle of knots, I'd gift myself the freedom to focus on the end rather than the means.

Back at Pitho Rooms, George, the hotelier, was setting crockery out on a breakfast bar. As I collected my plate, I asked if he knew of a taxi driver I could employ for the morning. A series of phone calls resulted in Kostas being hauled out of bed. He'd had a late night working his shift at a Delphi restaurant and had been looking forward to a lie-in, but he said he was glad of the opportunity to earn sixty euros. He would happily drive me to Distomo and the monastery, and I calculated that the time, fatigue and angst I'd save would be well worth the money. And, as he informed me within seconds of my climbing into the back seat of his car, I was lucky to find a driver who spoke such good English.

We stopped in the pretty ski resort town of Arahova so Kostas could pick up a much-needed iced coffee, but it didn't take long to get to Distomo. There was only one lonely, driverless taxi parked in the town square, and I murmured a 'thank you' to whichever Muse had guided me to abandon my blueprint for the day.

It was too early to visit the museum commemorating the massacre, so we headed straight to the monastery. The clean lines of this pleasing collection of Byzantine architecture emerged from a cloud of purple flowers as we approached. Overlooking a sweeping valley of olive groves, it was, according to the sign, 'still a vibrant monastic community with great vigor.'

It was here I saw the first of the three bodies of saints I would encounter in churches during this trip. Only one of Saint Luke's hands was exposed to the gaze of the faithful; a gossamer veil concealed his face, and snug black velvet slippers enclosed his feet.

In the past, when visiting colonial museums in my own country and around the world, I have pondered the ethics of putting people's bodies or body parts on show, even while acknowledging the strange fascination they exert. There's a great deal we can learn from the scientific study of those buried long ago, but exhibiting them has felt a step too far. If nothing else, it seems more than a coincidence that the displayers have often been white, while those I've seen on display have usually been people of colour. There were skeletons curled in huge clay pots in the storeroom of the museum where I worked in 1990s South Africa, and I used to wonder how those people's descendants might feel if they knew their ancestors lay in that dark, lonely warehouse. I would dip my head as I passed them, that tiny token of respect all I had to offer.

Here in Greece, though, the bodies of the dead were preserved by their own communities for the purpose of veneration. They weren't corpses plundered from their final resting places by outsiders and exhibited for the voyeurism of others. This was different. It was about reverence rather than exploitation.

One building led to another, until Kostas and I found ourselves in the crypt, standing before the tomb where the saint was previously interred. In sombre silence, we walked through a poppy-strewn courtyard to a building labelled '*Fotanamma*'. I asked Kostas what this word meant. He had no idea but, with a wry glance at the smoke-blackened walls, he said, 'It looks as if someone set fire to the place.'

A sign on the way out explained that the sooty walls were not the result of malicious arsonists. Instead, we read, the *fotanamma* was where: 'the monks gathered to warm themselves during cold nights. It is a room supported by columns and roofed with cylindrical vaults, with small ventilation openings for the smoke.'[2]

Kostas opened the front passenger door of his taxi for me. There was no question, now, of my sitting in the back, our chatting made awkward by the distance between us. I balanced his coffee cup on my lap while he drove to Distomo, and he told me he always felt at peace after spending time in such a holy place.

This peace was shattered at Distomo's museum.

The building's neat exterior of dressed stone and red roof tiles enclosed a disturbing display. Row upon row of black-and-white photographic portraits lined the walls. They were of the hundreds who had been slaughtered, as well as the three Nazi officers who had set the Distomo massacre in motion. Long lists of the victims' names and ages were evidence that the occupiers showed no mercy, killing even

---

2   In August 2023, just months before these pages went to print, wildfires swept large areas of Greece. Online newspapers reported that the oldest building in the Moni Osios Loukas complex was ablaze, and that a senior bishop, the Metropolitan of Thebes and Livadeia, wept as he battled the flames alongside crews of firefighters. Thankfully, no human lives were lost, and the relics were kept safe. One building was severely damaged by the fire, but it was reported that the walls could be restored and the destroyed roof could be replaced. In September, the monastery was once again open to the public.

the elderly and babies as young as two months. A floor-to-ceiling photograph showed shelves divided into 190 dark compartments, each housing a murdered skull.

Living, breathing people reduced to bare bones.

Having Kostas as my companion made the visit even more poignant than it would otherwise have been. He'd grown up on one of the Greek islands, but his father had been born in this region, and Kostas was visibly upset. A busload of German sightseers had visited the museum just ahead of us, and we talked about the value of people taking responsibility for traumatic aspects of their nation's history, and about how I experience this as a white South African who grew up under apartheid. About how awful it is that people whose company you might enjoy if you had met in a peacetime taverna could commit such ghastly atrocities during war. About how those infants killed would now have been in their seventies; their grandchildren would have been Kostas's colleagues and friends.

We got back to Delphi three minutes late for his noon shift at the restaurant. He assured me this wouldn't be a problem, even though he still had to change into his work clothes. I gave him a generous tip and appreciated it when he checked to be sure I had not misunderstood the price. Some of the buildings we'd visited at the monastery and some of what we had learned at the museum were new to him, too, and I hoped he'd got more out of the morning than some much-needed cash, that he'd found our conversations as interesting as I had.

I took a brief time-out in my room to clear my mind, and then set out for Delphi's main archaeological site to see the egg-shaped boulder marking the navel of the Earth, called the Omphalos, and the temple where Apollo's oracle made her far-reaching proclamations. Her prophecies — interpreted through skilful intermediaries who, no doubt, were serving powerful agendas of their own — affected decisions ranging from making laws to waging wars.

It's significant that the maxim 'Know Thyself' was once inscribed at the entrance to this temple, greeting pilgrims who'd come from afar. My own Greek journey of midlife self-discovery was, in literary terms, a trope that suffered from overuse. It was unsettling to recognise that my life story might be a platitude, but could the cliché — of travelling to a foreign land to find yourself — date back to ancient times? *If so, does that negate the power of my experience, or enhance it?*

Enhance it, I should think, but try as I might, I couldn't feel the magic in this part of Delphi. Two days into the trip, my body was still feeling the effects of the long flight. Although my headache had disappeared, the muscle that ran from my neck down to my left shoulder had clenched into a tight knot. Plus, moving from monastery to massacre site had drained my emotions and wrung me dry. I was exhausted, and grateful not to be sitting on the highway outside Distomo, anxiously hoping to flag down a fast-moving bus. My afternoon visit turned out to be one of interest, rather than the enchantment that had cast its allure over my illicit early-morning moments alone in the Sanctuary of Athena Pronaia.

Nevertheless, I was determined to visit every part of the site, and I trudged all the way to the stadium. It was a gruelling uphill slog, and how the athletes had any breath left to compete in their games has to be one of the mysteries of Ancient Greece. My Fitbit recorded 21,531 steps for the day, with a gradient equal to 88 flights of stairs — most of those were on the slow trek up to the stadium.

That night, I sat on my little balcony sipping wine and eating a takeaway pita souvlaki I'd bought for the princely sum of two euros. Jeffrey Siger's *Devil of Delphi*, a rollicking whodunnit set amid the landmarks of the region, had me engrossed. Siger's police detective books always make for an engaging read, but what I love about them is his enviable sense of place. When I came to a pivotal scene set in Moni Osios Loukas, with a deeply flawed villain hiding in the crypt while a furtive figure lurked outside, I smiled. The shady character was skulking in the same courtyard scattered with poppies through which we had strolled that morning.

CHAPTER FIVE
DELPHI TO CORFU

O NE OF THE THINGS I've learned about Greece is that it is sometimes simpler to return to Athens and fly to your next destination, rather than travel over land and sea by public transportation. This is a pity. I would have preferred to experience the landscape through the windows of a train — or even a bus — than to squander time in an airport queue, but neither my guidebook nor my kind hotel hosts could suggest a more manageable route. To get from Delphi to the island of Kerkyra, known to English-speakers as Corfu, I'd have to backtrack to the capital and catch a plane.

On the road to Athens, I kept my eyes peeled for that strange, matte-black church that had made such an impression on me as we sped past it a few days before, but it eluded me. I wonder, now, if it ever existed.

~ ~ ~

Corfu was famously the 1930s stomping ground of the Durrell family, so I gave Gerald Durrell's *My Family and Other Animals* another go. After all, the British television show *The Durrells*, about the four years they lived on the island, was good fun. I hoped my tastes might have changed enough, in the three decades since I'd first slid the paperback from my father's shelves, to enjoy it this time around. Despite Durrell's beautifully crafted prose in the opening pages, though, I couldn't get into the story. Wondering how much my irrational fear of creepy crawlies had to do with my inability to lose myself in the great naturalist's childhood memoir, which seemed to feature an inordinate number of bugs, I closed it after a few chapters and opened the last book of Sulari Gentill's Hero Trilogy instead.

I had fallen in love with Gentill's work through her Rowland Sinclair series of historical mysteries set partly in Sydney between the two World Wars. As a new Australian, I had known nothing of the rise of fascism in 1930s Australia, or the drama that accompanied the inauguration of the Sydney Harbour Bridge, until I read her stories. Her Hero books are quite different, and I might never have picked them up if my local indie bookseller hadn't recommended them for my first expedition to Greece. They retell the events of Homer's *The Iliad* and *The Odyssey* and Virgil's *The Aeneid* from a fantastical young adult perspective.

By the time I got to the Bella Venezia, my hotel on the outskirts of Corfu's World Heritage Old Town, even the offer of a welcome drink couldn't dilute my weariness. I turned it down. All I wanted was to take a shower and then collapse into bed with a book. When the cheerful lady at reception said there was a complimentary bottle of wine in my room, and then presented me with a glossy booklet on the history of the Grand Hotel d'Angleterre et Belle Venise, as it was formerly known, I was quite content.

Opening the cover, I read: 'Noble and kind traveller, here you are in the land of the Phaeacians. King Odysseus first stopped at our beautiful island while on his way back to Ithaca.'

Wait a minute! Wasn't the land of the Phaeacians one of the settings in *Chasing Odysseus*, the first book of Gentill's trilogy? I grabbed my e-reader to check. Sure enough, there it was. And wasn't the magical boat the protagonists were still sailing in Book Three a Phaeacian craft? Yes, she was.

Quite by chance, I had arrived on the very island about which I'd been reading. I'd heard claims that Corfu was the setting for William Shakespeare's play, *The Tempest*. But I'd no idea that this land might once have been the legendary home of *The Odyssey*'s Nausicaa — a name which looks far more like a seasick character in an Asterix and Obelix graphic novel, than the lovely young princess described by Homer.

~ ~ ~

Setting out early, I passed a tribute to novelist Lawrence Durrell, Gerald's older brother, whose home I had stumbled upon on Rhodes the year before. His gruff face looked out from the embossed metal plaque, his shiny nose golden from the eager touch of tourists. Below him were the words, 'Greece is the country that offers you the discovery of yourself.'

I mulled this over, thinking of how the mood of this Grecian journey was already so different from the previous year's, and how this change reflected my altered state of mind. Last September, mired in the after-effects of my Sri Lankan bus accident, I'd embarked on a desperate quest to seek the passion of my youth; I'd needed an adventure to rescue myself from the doldrums of my own middlescence. Any dissatisfaction with my lot thawed in the summer heat of that trip's joyous escapades. It melted away, finally, on my hike along Santorini's caldera, where I came to grips with my own privilege. This springtime journey, by contrast, was one of gentle gladness rather than sharp-edged exhilaration. I was slowing down, relinquishing control, indulging in the humble pleasures of the senses.

Rambling along broad promenades and narrow lanes, I visited Corfu's Old Fortress, where I climbed the long way around to the lighthouse, and the New Fortress, where I encountered a head-bopping lizard atop a sunny stone wall. I came across a world-class museum of Asian art housed, somewhat surprisingly, in the grand old British colonial Palace of Saint Michael and Saint George. Then, standing in a lengthy line of people waiting to file through the cramped chamber behind the altar of a church, I paid my respects to the body of Agios Spyridon, who died in the fourth century. His relics lay in an ornate silver casket, his neck bent at an awkward angle, as devotees bowed first over his velvet slippers and then over his exposed face. A monk chanted in a melodious baritone in the corner of the room, pausing only to urge a woman, over-zealous in her adoration, to move along and allow others a chance to pay homage to the saint.

I explored the old town and the new, exulting in the kaleidoscope of fresh produce at market stalls and nipping into a boutique to buy a funky new daypack, a beachy number striped in shades of blue and cream, complete with buckles and canvas straps. This would stand in for the faithful bag Megan had gifted me, now a casualty to a broken zipper, until I could have it repaired.

A poster in a shop window caused me a comical double-take, and I had to triple-check that I'd interpreted the Greek letters correctly. It advertised a theatrical production of *Don Camillo*, based on the novels written by Giovannino Guareschi in the aftermath of the Second World War. These humorous stories relate the political wrangles between an Italian priest and his village's communist mayor, both ex-partisans, who are fiery adversaries and — when it really matters — friends.

Stunned by the personal serendipity of the moment, I posted a photograph on social media:

> 29 May 2017
> My dad had a shelf filled with *Don Camillo* books, and, despite our ideological differences, I enjoyed them too. I hadn't thought of the books in years, maybe decades, until a few weeks ago in Australia, when Adam dragged me into yet another charity shop and I found a battered old edition, which I bought for a couple of dollars.

~ ~ ~

It was a day of tiny churches and azure views, but my most agreeable find by far was the Casa Parlante, billed as a living history museum. Its A-frame sign, perched on the sidewalk, promised, 'History of Corfu is being revived in a 19th century noble mansion. Moving human figures, scents and sounds, all invite you to a travel back in time.'

A young woman named Fani welcomed me inside. In near-perfect, prettily accented English, she escorted me from one room filled with fine period furnishings to the next. Her single slip, when she called a low lintel a doorstep, was endearing. 'Lintel' is a delightful word describing the crossbeam above a doorway, but there are plenty of first-language English speakers who wouldn't be familiar with its use. Her unintentional inversion of its meaning reminded me of a long-ago moment in a Sri Lankan hospital, when morphine had turned my world upside down. Lying flat on my back as orderlies pushed my gurney through a labyrinth of hospital corridors, I perceived each approaching lintel as an obstacle in our path — something very like a doorstep — and braced for a bump. Each time the wheels passed smoothly through a doorway, the morphine haze was tinged with a sense of wonder.

The automated mannequins standing in for the mansion's erstwhile residents recalled me to the present. They were awkward, even a bit creepy, but they made an eye-catching counterpoint to Fani's commentary. While the mistress of the house raised a cup of tea to her lips in a series of uncomfortable jerks, Fani graciously offered me a glass of traditional kumquat liqueur. The patriarch perused his newspaper in the study while, in the bedroom, Mary applied her feather duster to the polished furniture in rough, robotic strokes.

Mary was a servant of the wealthy people who lived here, and, if Fani's stories were anything to go by, she had good reason to feel resentful. Not only did she have to carry the family's toilet waste two kilometres to empty it into the sea, she also had to delay ironing their bedsheets until evening. The freshly pressed linen would warm her mistress's bed, while Mary herself rode a donkey home in the wintry night air.

Grandmother rocked in her chair by the window. The children, their governess and the cook were all present, and the insights into their lives were fascinating. Fani, who speaks four languages, balanced her knowledgeable delivery with good humour, filling the rooms with tales of nineteenth-century Corfiot history and culture.

Tired out from the day's explorations, I returned to the Bella Venezia, a hotel a tad more upmarket than my usual accommodations. With this trip organised on such short notice, I hadn't had time to shop around for more frugal options, but the price was more than fair by Australian standards. And I appreciated the extra touches: the complimentary wine, the souvenir booklet, and the daily magnificence of the breakfast buffet. This boasted Greek yoghurt from Ioannina, which I drizzled with pure Corfiot honey and ate with enormous red strawberries, handmade jams and marmalades with fresh bread and butter, and slices of sesame-encrusted minced fig preserve. These added a sweet edge to the variety of cheeses and cold meats including *graviera* and *noumboulo*, organic olives and feta from the Peloponnese, and an egg station I never had the capacity to visit. *Mandoles*, a Corfiot speciality, were caramelised almonds and my favourite, and there was as much fresh-squeezed orange juice as I could drink. After the breakfast room closed, though, the hotel's food was limited to bar snacks.

That evening, I decided not to venture out to a restaurant. Instead, I relaxed in the courtyard with a gin and tonic and a ham-and-cheese toastie, the most substantial item on the menu, and read up on the next day's excursion. My guidebook had tipped me off that Albania was just a short boat ride away, so I'd booked a spot on a tour that would visit the World Heritage Site of Butrint and a freshwater spring called the Blue Eye.

CHAPTER SIX
A DAY IN ALBANIA

THERE'S NOTHING QUITE LIKE the thrill of crossing a
border for the first time — and if the crossing is by
boat, that thrill is tinged with romance. For Europeans,
international travel is a hop, skip and jump away, but for those
of us living on the east coast of Australia, or raised near the
southern tip of Africa, travel to another country has always
been a significant undertaking. And Albania is a land about
which I knew nothing; its name conjured only a vague image
of Soviet-bloc bleakness.

My passport received an exit stamp from Greece but there
was no one waiting to ink its pages when we reached Sarandë on
the Albanian shore. This was the thirty-second country I'd had
the privilege of visiting but, despite it not being a member of the
European Union, it left no memento in my travel document.

A tour guide herded us off the ferry and straight onto
a claustrophobic coach. Her running commentary raced
our route, repeating each snippet of information in three

languages. The droning voice sped up as we approached the next landmark to flash past our windows, then slowed as the bus decelerated into the curves of the hills that climbed out of the town.

I surrendered my autonomy as our shuttle weaved through the greens and blues of farmland and waterways. This excursion, booked on a whim, would be the kind of package tourism experience I usually avoided at all costs. The romance was evaporating, but the landscape was far from bleak.

Butrint National Park is a sprawling tapestry of wetlands and forests, with the ruins of four ancient civilisations — Hellenistic, Roman, Byzantine and Venetian — stitched across its surface. To safeguard the fabric of its woodland habitats, archaeologists have set aside large areas of the park where they refrain from unpicking the threads of history.

In fact, the entire park balances a delicate compromise between natural and cultural heritage management. The sacred sanctuary of Asclepius — established as a centre of healing in the fourth century BCE — is sinking, millimetre by slow millimetre, into a khaki pool colonised by frogs and miniature turtles. At the graceful sixth-century circular baptistery, in contrast, the floor is covered to protect it from the elements. A signboard showed its design, concentric mosaic rings pierced by pillars like broken teeth, and explained:

... seasonal rise and fall of the water level in the surrounding lagoon results in repeated submerging and drying of the pavement. If the mosaic were constantly exposed to the air this process would lead rapidly to permanent and irreversible deterioration. So, to ensure the long-term preservation of the mosaics, the floor of the Baptistery will normally have to be kept covered. Every few years the mosaics will be uncovered for a limited period to allow public access and scientific conservation.

My travels and reading had brought me to a point where I could see connections all around me, even here in Albania. When I'd first set foot on Balkan soil, I relied on a mishmash of half-remembered mythology and popular culture references to make sense of what I encountered. Now, everything seemed to fit together as neatly as that pattern of tiny tiles that once circled the baptistery's font of holy water.

As we'd approached Butrint, we had passed a signpost pointing to one of the infamous Ali Pasha's early-nineteenth-century fortifications, accessible only by boat. Ali Pasha was the son of Khamco, a woman who, after her husband's death, took up arms and captained a gang of bandits. She was ambushed by rival bands and taken prisoner, along with her adolescent son and daughter. They were brutalised by their captors and, after their ransom, Ali became a vengeful warlord. Through marriage and political intrigue, he rose to the position of Ottoman governor of Ioannina, a Greek town just forty kilometres away from the present-day border with Albania. Eventually, his lust for power brought him into disfavour with the Sultan, and he was assassinated in 1822.

When I first came across traces of Ali Pasha's story, while exploring the iconic Greek site of Meteora in 2016, I read that he was also called *Aslan*, 'the Lion' in Turkish. That was where I learned of his efforts to quell the rebellion of the Greeks against their Ottoman invaders. I might never have heard of Ali's mother — a woman of Amazonian courage, albeit with a troubling moral compass — if the linguistic link with *The Chronicles of Narnia* hadn't sent me to Google to find out more. Now, our proximity to his stronghold underlined the historical ties between Albania and Greece during the era of the Ottoman Empire.

This wasn't the only connection I stumbled across at Butrint. In a Venetian castle at the top of a hill, a familiar name on an exhibition panel clicked a new tile into place. This was a setting in the very book I'd cracked open a couple of days before: the site of a new colony where Hector's widow, Andromache, and his brother, Helenus, were exiled from defeated Troy.

I wish I could say I was familiar with this chapter of the Trojans' story from the pages of *The Aeneid*, in which

Aeneas sails from Phaeacia to Buthrotum — or, in modern terminology, from Corfu to Butrint. Actually, it was Aussie author Sulari Gentill's *The Blood of Wolves* that gifted me this nexus with legends that were already ancient when Virgil put pen to papyrus two thousand years ago. Of course, as *The Aeneid* is set roughly twelve centuries BCE, and the oldest ruins I saw dated to the sixth century BCE, I still had to use my imagination to picture the scene faced by Gentill's (oops, I mean Virgil's) characters when they made landfall here. I went out on a limb and tagged Gentill in a Facebook photograph of the site, and was ecstatic when she liked my post.

Motoring away from Butrint, our coach passed the only evidence of Soviet-bloc bleakness I would see in Albania: dome-shaped bunkers at the side of the road. These were a relic from the Cold War, when the government urged the population to construct defensive shelters. In an echo of the hysteria gripping the West, they built around 200,000 of these concrete bunkers in preparation for an attack that never came.

Our group paused for a meal on a second-floor restaurant terrace, but we leaned over the balcony when we heard hoots and yells. A motorcade of cheering youth was driving through town, their lithe bodies perched half outside the car windows as they laughed and waved T-shirts. 'Today,' our guide explained, repeating herself in English, French and German, 'they finish school. Tomorrow, they will study for their exams.'

Lunch over, we headed to our next stop: an exquisite pool of startling aquamarine. The source of the remarkably clear Bistricë River, the Blue Eye's water bubbles up at a staggering rate — often approaching 18,400 litres per second — from a spring more than fifty metres deep. Exactly how deep is a conundrum, as the force of the water prevents divers from plumbing its depths. At its surface, though, the pool is a peaceful playground for dragonflies. Myriad sparks of iridescent blue hover above the turquoise ripples and dart among the greenery, silent against the gushing soundtrack of the current that surges out of the earth.

After filling my drinking bottle from the pool, the water's chill a shock against my fingers, I tried to capture these flying gems on film. It was a laughing game of catch, their fluttering wings far too quick for my camera's lens to grab, and the footage does little justice to the beauty of their dance.

~ ~ ~

In Sarandë, our guide gave us an hour and a half to wander before catching our ferry to Greece. The day had lifted my spirits in ways I hadn't foreseen when I'd boarded that bus filled with sunburnt adults and bickering children. Still, I relished the freedom of an unaccompanied amble through the sleepy town after being cooped for hours in a packed coach.

A supermarket gave me a pretext to break away from the group. The errand would have been a weak excuse without a purchase to bolster my cover, so I bought a bottle of brandy for my hosts at my next destination. It was cheap at a few euros, but our guide had assured us that Skënderbeu *konjak* was 'very famous under communism' and it might make a good little gift with this tagline behind it.

At the harbour, I caught up with the cluster of tourists from our bus — all loud voices and peeling shoulders — browsing at a row of souvenir stands selling sunglasses and beaded necklaces. I made off in the opposite direction, where a long, paved promenade led out of sight of the line of market stalls to a small beach. A couple of sunbathers lay motionless in separate solitude, while four boys, ranging in age from about six to twelve years, paddled at the water's edge. A hundred metres ahead was a swimming zone, surrounded on three sides by tiered seating. On the fourth, it was open to the sea and a collection of boats clinking at their moorings.

I didn't go quite that far. Instead, I chose a spot on the beach, with a jetty to my left and a children's play area at my back. I'd been wearing my swimsuit under my clothes all day in the futile hope that the Blue Eye would turn out to be a swimming hole, so I seized on this unexpected opportunity for a solo dip. I peeled off my loose-fitting blouse, shawl and skirt, and inched barefoot across the sharp pebbles. As I waded into the sea, a welcome breeze riffled across my damp skin.

The boys found my careful steps into the water hilarious, and the youngest child just about collapsed with glee when I dunked my head under the salty surface. The cause of their extreme amusement was a mystery — it was unlikely to be my modest one-piece, as they showed no interest in the bikini-clad woman sunning herself nearby — but I laughed along with them anyway. There was a half-submerged soda bottle bobbing in the tide, and they called to me to retrieve it. At least, that's what I thought they wanted; we shared no language. I swam out to the plastic bottle and discovered it was half-filled with sand, its lid screwed on tight, its heft making it easy to toss to them on the shore.

When I emerged from the water, the boys showed off for me. Climbing on the playground equipment, they shouted to me to photograph them and then ran over, giggling, to look at the images on my phone. The pictures burst with energetic fun, the boys' bright, toothy grins contrasting with their grubby jeans and tracksuit pants. My younger self would have shared the photos without a thought. Our world isn't as innocent as the spontaneous play of children, though. Over decades of travel, I've grown mindful about not publishing snaps of minors without the consent of their parents.

My day in Albania ended with high-fives from the kids followed by a stroll past the foundations of a fifth-century synagogue, while a muezzin called the faithful to prayer in a rich tenor that rolled out over the city and the Ionian Sea beyond.

~ ~ ~

What struck me on the ferry back to Corfu, my head filled with the heroes of antiquity, was how close these lands are to each other. Whenever I'd imagined the events of *The Odyssey*, I'd pictured great ocean voyages with sea-weary sailors trapped aboard ship for months, desperate for the scarce sight of solid ground. And some of the islands mentioned in these tales are indeed remote. But what you can see between Corfu — the land of the Phaeacians visited by Greek wanderers after the battle of Troy — and Butrint — settled by a band of Trojan exiles — is a sea speckled with islets. At all times, you are in view of more than one oasis of green or brown breaking the surface of the cerulean waters. Some are small outcrops, but others are large enough to be habitable. A substantial part of the decade-long Odyssey may have been a matter of hopping from one nearby isle to the next.

As for me? That despised tourist bus had been the vessel to take me to new lands. It had transported me to wonders I'd never otherwise have seen, and allowed me a few perfect moments on an Albanian shore. *From now on*, I resolved, *I'll be a lot less snobbish about the dreaded group tour.*

In my hotel room, a new book prepared me for a mental shift forward of more than three thousand years, as well as a geographical shift to my next port of call, just two days away. The novel was one of my all-time favourites, *Captain Corelli's Mandolin* by Louis de Bernières. The story is set on the island of Kefalonia, but the line I remembered most clearly made no mention of Greece: 'He says that in Ireland it rains every day and that in Chile there's a desert where it has never rained at all.'

The first time I read those words was in 1999, on a damp, grey day in the Irish countryside. I had just moved, heartbroken, from a year in Chile, where I had visited the Atacama Desert with the man I'd believed would become my husband. Now, rereading the book in Greece, I came across a reference to the saint whose venerated remains I'd visited in the church of Agios Spyridon the day before. I drifted off, filled with the glow of literary wanderlust.

CHAPTER SEVEN
CORFU TO KEFALONIA

BOARDING A BUS WAS less of a conscious challenge, now, and one of the local blue buses could take me to Mon Repos, a little south of Corfu Town.

My *Lonely Planet* had recommended the estate for its wooded parklands, museum and ancient ruins, and the spruiker for a tourist hop-on-hop-off coach had done me the unwitting favour of preparing me to come equipped for a swim. She'd been trying, unsuccessfully, to sell me a ticket for the coach. It wouldn't stop at Mon Repos, even though it drove right past the estate. 'But,' she said, with a dismissive flick of her hair, 'there is nothing there. Only a place to swim. And there are many other places for swimming.'

The conflicting information left me unsure of whether Mon Repos would be worth a visit, but the number 2A bus got me there easily. It was surprisingly close to the city; it would have taken only half an hour to walk if I'd been sure of the way.

The bus dropped me beside the graceful ruins of a church, signposted as the 'Palaiopolis Archaeological Site'. I skirted the fence until I got to the entrance, but it was clear it had been padlocked shut for a very long time. Behind the metal palings, a boardwalk sagged around the ruin. Its warped boards were loose, missing or splintered.

Across the road stood another archaeological site, this one protected by shade sails, also behind a locked gate. As I stepped forward to photograph the site and its distant signboards, hoping the zoom lens would allow me to decipher their text, I stumbled into a shallow hole in the ground. Not my first time! And not the deepest, by far. Still, I lost both my balance and my battle with gravity, and I was lucky not to sprain an ankle. There were no lasting injuries, not even to my pride as there was nobody around to witness my fall.

I limped into the Mon Repos estate and made my way along shady paths to a gracious manor. Once the summer residence of British governors, it was later owned by Greek royalty, until the republican government exiled them and confiscated the building. It was the birthplace of Prince Philip, born to the royal family of Greece and Denmark. Said to have been birthed on a dining table and smuggled out of Greece in a fruit crate as a toddler, he grew up to marry Elizabeth, then heir to the throne of the United Kingdom and a dozen other lands. The mansion now houses a small but interesting museum with displays on archaeology, art and the lifestyle of those who first lived there.

A collection of nineteenth-century photographs of Corfu hung in a side room. Many were taken from the same vantage points where I'd snapped my shots two days before, and the déjà vu was staggering. The photographer was a young British major named John Shakespear (without the third e). He had come to the island in 1856 after serving in the Crimean War, and had stayed next door to my hotel. So, too, had humorous nonsense poet Edward Lear — he of 'The Owl and the Pussycat' and 'The Jumblies' fame — who was brought to life as a young ornithological illustrator in a book I'd read recently, Melissa Ashley's *The Birdman's Wife*.

Upstairs, a shiny cache of minuscule silver coins snagged my attention: 510 of them spilling from a broken clay pot. Archaeologists had unearthed them in the nearby ancient agora, or marketplace, and dated them to the third century BCE. You have to wonder about the traders who had hoarded these coins. How long did it take them to accumulate this treasure? Why were they saving their money? And what calamity resulted in it being lost through the ages?

There was also a scale model of Corfu that awakened a childlike joy in me. I pushed its buttons, each lighting up a specific area on the miniature reproduction of the estate, and tried to memorise which way I should go next.

Leaving the museum, I followed a path that soon became a dangerously eroded track slipping towards the sea. Worn brick steps peeked out from drifts of dead leaves, making it clear this had once been a well-used pathway, so I persevered. After I'd climbed through two tangles of branches, though, the trail came to an abrupt end in a treacherous sand-slide slithering down the cliff to the ocean below. I retraced my cautious way to the museum, where, if I had just taken the time to look around on exiting the building, I would have seen a sign pointing the route to the Doric temple.

Deciding to wait until a noisy group of primary schoolkids moved out of earshot, I settled onto a bench sandwiched between a paddock and the ruins of a small church. On a barely legible page, torn from a notebook and stuck to a faded board, red handwritten letters proclaimed: 'DO NOT FEED THE HORSES!!!' As I bit into an apricot filched from that morning's breakfast table, savouring its sour tartness, an optimistic pony stared at me from one side and a curious kitten, interrupted from its play on the chapel roof, from the other.

Thankfully, the children weren't heading to the temple. I passed their flustered teacher trying to hold their attention in the shade of a sycamore tree, and continued on until I caught sight of shattered columns in a tranquil location below the path.

Someone had broken the flimsy wooden barrier that had once blocked off the slope leading to the temple, and a couple of tentative steps brought me to the edge. There was an easy way down, and I felt an urge to wander the overgrown ruins like an explorer of old, alone except for the tiny yellow butterflies fluttering above the weeds. But this site hadn't been set up for visitors. While my careful footsteps were unlikely to do much damage, the tread of innumerable tourists, of whom I was merely one, would surely leave its mark on the ancient remains. I may have climbed that gate in Delphi, but that was when I was certain my doing so could cause no harm. And, even though that early-morning ramble was precious, a niggle of guilt worried away at the logic of my self-justification. This time, I resisted the temptation and turned away.

Then I found the 'place to swim'.

A long stone pier, occupied by a dozen or so teenagers, stretched into the sea. I wondered if the Greek school year aligned with that of nearby Albania, and if these students had opted to celebrate the first day of their study break together, here at this sunny cove, rather than bent over their books alone at home. The boys were running along the pier and plunging into the water in noisy camaraderie. The girls ignored them, sunning themselves and chatting, although I have no doubt they were excruciatingly aware of the boys' every move. I remember that dance from my own adolescence.

I picked my way along the mulch-covered sand until I came to a shady patch, where I read a couple more chapters of

Captain Corelli's Mandolin before wading into the crisp water for a swim. The splashing games of the teenagers made a happy backdrop to the peace of the beach, and they didn't disturb my rest.

Not yet ready to catch the bus into town, I left the estate parkland and 'followed my nose' — as my grandmother used to say — down a road to see where it might go. I hoped it would take me to another temple, but I'd misremembered the museum model and gone in the wrong direction. By the time I realised I was making my way along that morning's bus route, I'd walked halfway to my hotel. I decided to keep going into the centre of Corfu Town.

My mission for the afternoon was to find the synagogue and the memorial to the two thousand Corfiot Jews who were taken to the concentration camps during the Second World War. To my frustration, even though a map showed I was on the right road to the synagogue, both landmarks eluded me.

Dog-tired, I shifted focus. Retreating up the same road to escape the tourist-thronged waterfront, I spotted a souvlaki shop. It's not often I want a beer — maybe once or twice a year — but today was one of those days. I wolfed down a pita souvlaki with a chilled Alfa lager for just four euros, including a tip. Hunger tamed, I resumed my search and located the synagogue a couple of minutes later.

This airy house of worship, with its open windows and pastel-painted walls, lifted my spirits. The respite was heartening but brief, ending when I picked up a photocopied pamphlet. Its smudged text outlined the bones of a grim story.

The Corfiot Jewish community totalled somewhere between five and seven thousand people towards the end of the nineteenth century. In 1891, everything changed. An ugly lie tore through the island. The rumour was horrendous: that Jews had killed a Christian girl in ritual sacrifice and used her blood in the baking of Passover bread. The little girl, called Rubina and only eight years old, had indeed been murdered. But she was Jewish, and her death was a tragedy, not a ritual.

The resultant violent hysteria, whipped up by bigots and exploited by opportunists, led to an exodus of Jews seeking a safer life elsewhere. Two thousand were still on Corfu in the early twentieth century, and that's roughly how many the Gestapo shipped to the death camps just a year before the war ended. Fewer than 150 Corfiot Jews survived.

Today, the pamphlet told me, the Jews living on Corfu number around sixty.

I'd given up on finding the memorial statue. Although my guidebook had mentioned it, I hadn't seen it marked on any map. As so often happens, though, I stumbled upon it soon after I abandoned my quest. It portrayed a woman clutching her baby, her hand raised in a futile attempt to ward off danger, and a boy leaning against his father in despair. Its rough stone plinth bore plaques in Greek and English:

NEVER AGAIN FOR ANY NATION
Dedicated to the memory of the 2000 Jews of
Corfu who perished in the Nazi concentration
camps of Auschwitz and Birkenau in June 1944

I headed to my hotel in a sombre mood — conscious of
how petty the trifling hunger and fatigue I'd felt earlier had
been, compared with true suffering — and turned in for an
early night.

~ ~ ~

As our plane climbed into the skies above Corfu the next
day, I looked down and picked out the Mon Repos swimming
spot, identifiable by the long pier pointing out to sea like an
index finger. It appeared as peaceful from the air as it had on
the beach.

Soon, I was peering at the mainland from the window of the
smallest plane in which I'd ever travelled. It had the capacity to
hold up to thirty passengers, one flight attendant and, I hoped
with every fibre of my being, two pilots. My standard-size
laptop backpack wouldn't fit in the tiny space under the single
seat in front of me, and there were no overhead compartments.
I'd have been happy to hold the bag on my lap, but the flight
attendant moved me across the aisle to a vacant double seat
near the rear of the plane, where I could strap it in beside me.

The journey took place in two legs: from Corfu to Preveza on the mainland, the flying time was fifteen minutes; from Preveza to the island of Kefalonia, it took twenty. Greece from the air is utterly lovely, with its sweeping greenery and majestic mountains, its white-fringed coves and vast curving bays. I was a bit distracted, though. Air turbulence feels much more personal in a plane this size.

~ ~ ~

There are few kinder services you can offer a traveller than to wash a load of their dirty laundry. I'd come across a laundromat on Corfu, but it was closed. Here on Kefalonia, where I'd moved into the downstairs flat beneath the home of my book-club friend Kate's parents, they gave me the gift of clean clothes. I found myself pegging wet garments on an outdoor washing line for the first time in years.

At home in Australia, our apartment building's strict rules prohibit hanging anything on the balconies. We drape wet clothes on the backs of chairs and from hangers hooked over the wooden rails of our four-poster bed. The bed was one of Adam's impulsive eBay purchases and looks ridiculously over-the-top in our little flat, but I've grown to love it. And it pays its way when it comes to getting our washing dry.

Now, I was hanging laundry amid fruit trees and birdsong, filled with joy at the rich colours and scents and the warmth of sunlight on my skin in the cooling evening. How had this ever seemed a chore?

My hosts, Linda and Paul, had brought me olives and wine, a corkscrew that I remembered how to use on the second go — most Australian wineries use screw tops — and their Wi-Fi password. For the first time on this trip, I settled at my laptop.

When I first came to Greece, I thought it was excitement and freedom that were missing from my existence, and that it was travel itself that had the potential to make my life extraordinary. What I discovered, though, was what I needed: to recognise my own privilege and find contentment in what I had. I fell back in love with my life.

I confronted my dread of road travel and found my wanderlust but, while I revelled in the accomplishments and exhilarations of the journey, my subconscious took me a step further. It enfolded the passion to write within the cloth of a dream, and bestowed it on me like a blessing.

~ ~ ~

My writing that evening stimulated unexpected memories.

The last time I'd hung laundry outdoors had been four years earlier, in Naples.

Megan, my closest friend, had persuaded me to meet her in Europe. This was to be her first overseas trip, one she was taking to achieve a major goal on her bucket list: attending the Belgian Grand Prix. When she first asked me to join her in Paris, en route to Belgium, I surprised myself as much as anyone else by turning her down. Because I was still boarding planes to other cities in Australia, taking a budget Pacific cruise or two, and flying home to Cape Town every three years, I hadn't yet figured out that I was shrinking from adventurous travel. Let alone why, when everyone knew that travel was My Thing.

After months of coaxing, she convinced me. My only condition was that I'd visit the World Heritage town of Bruges while she watched the cars roar past on the Spa-Francorchamps circuit. For two glorious weeks, we travelled together through four countries. In Venice, we separated so she could see more deafening cars in Milan before returning to South Africa.

I went on to meet up with another important woman in my life. What Megan is to me, Shauna is to my sister Jenny: high school best friends who have stayed with us through the decades. Both Megan and Shauna have become part of my family over the years, very like sisters. They've never met, but both have been with me through some of my lowest points. Shauna was then going through a harrowing time of her own, after the heart-wrenching loss of her mother and sister in a traffic accident.

Shauna lives in Ireland and agreed to meet me for three days in Prague, but first I tested myself with a brief solo expedition: two nights in gritty Naples. I chose this city so I could visit Pompeii and nearby Herculaneum, the first-century towns that were simultaneously destroyed and conserved by the most famous eruption of Mount Vesuvius. My mum had visited Pompeii years before, and I wanted to walk in her footsteps.

I stayed in a grubby hostel where, at forty-one, I was the oldest guest by far. They had a washing machine, but no tumble dryer. Instead, I had to brave my fear of heights to lean out over a balcony railing, hanging wet clothes on lines strung above the heads of the pedestrians walking along the street seven storeys below. I needed both hands to manage the task, and my damaged left arm had never felt so close to betraying me.

~ ~ ~

I paused, my fingers hovering over the keyboard, before reaching for my mother's diary. Something had just clicked in my mind: Mum's visit to Pompeii would have taken place earlier on the same 1978 trip that included her stay in Greece. I must have read about it as I flicked through the pages, but I hadn't had any reason to focus on that entry. Until now.

Her journal — in typical, delightfully frustrating fashion — includes nothing about the archaeological site itself. Instead, it offers a loose collection of observations:

Date Thursday 5th
Place Rome Pompeii Naples Sorrento
Weather Gloomy — cloudy, rain at night
... Onto Pompeii for lunch. Michael's pasta!
Marias wine bottle. old man with accordion. Grans
worm. Bought post cards + book. Old lady with
medals. Franco 32 our guide. with purse. Madge
fell. Ice-cream with cucumber. Old lady in toilet.
2 oranges R1. old lady wanted Mom's umbrella.

So that's *where Madge fell over!* I thought, remembering
Madge's accident-prone antics from the first time I read
Mum's diary. *And I don't know who that 'old lady' was, but she
sure sounds like an interesting character.*

My mum's day-jaunt from Rome also included a stop
in Naples, which she described as 'very depressing + over
crowded'. She noted that she stayed in Room 101 at Rome's
Hotel delle Muse, and there was a definite itch in my travelling
feet as I located the hotel online. It was still in business.

~ ~ ~

My efforts to catch the next morning's phantom bus proved
to be most productive.

Rumour had it there would be an 8.30 a.m. bus to Argostoli
from Svoronata, where I was staying, so I got to the stop early,

guessing that village timetables might be inaccurate. I used the wait well, re-memorising the Greek numbers, which I had forgotten since my last trip, up to twenty. After a half-hour wait, an elderly Greek woman trudged past, pointed at her watch, and said, 'Bus. Eleven.' So, off I went to fill two hours exploring the area. I strolled from one end of Ai Helis beach to the other, then meandered down another unsealed road until I came across an incongruously large and ugly hotel.

On impulse, I entered and asked if it happened to be a pick-up point for any group excursions. I tend to avoid coach tours, but I'd had a good time on my day trip to Albania and, with local buses being few and far between, this might be the only way I could get around this sizeable island. My Kefalonian wish list included Melissani Cave Lake (because my friend Rebecca had shown me a captivating video clip), Fiskardo (one of the few towns on Kefalonia to survive the catastrophic 1953 earthquakes relatively unscathed), and the nearby island of Ithaca (I couldn't miss the chance to set foot on land once ruled by Odysseus). The hotel concierge was able to book tours visiting all these and more.

I made it back to the bus stop with twenty minutes to spare. This time, I didn't have to wait alone, reciting strings of numbers. An older Scottish couple were also waiting for the bus. Although I say 'older', they didn't have much more than a decade on me. Somehow, we were all getting old enough to chat wistfully about international options for retirement.

My plan was to retire with Adam in Cape Town in a couple of decades, if I couldn't work out a way to return before then. My new Scottish friends fancied retiring here in Greece sometime rather sooner. They hailed from a small town in Scotland called Biggar, and they were very much hoping 'Biggar won't get any bigger.' They told me about its historical connections to William Wallace and Mary, Queen of Scots, and then asked about my ancestors' countries of origin.

This is not a question I often get. Instead, in Australia, people are inclined to ask, 'So, are you British or Dutch?' I answer, sometimes a bit brusquely, that I am South African.

I told the Scottish couple my forebears came from many lands. The earliest South African Smith in our family was William, who came from England in 1820. But, I explained, the ancestor about whom we knew the most was my German great-great-grandmother, Marie Charlotte von Gropp. Orphaned as a toddler and sent to live with an abusive uncle, she went on to lead a most extraordinary life. She lived on four continents, sometimes in brutal poverty, enduring the hardships of nineteenth-century travel and the deaths of all but one of her eight children. She left behind an account of her life, handwritten on the back pages of a boarding house ledger. English was her second language, and her writing is riddled with eccentric spelling and grammar.

Grandma Gropp's memoir included an enchanting description of the four months she lived in the city she called Constantinople, once the Greek town of Byzantium and now a vibrant metropolis labelled on modern maps as Istanbul. Constantinople was arguably the most significant Greek Orthodox site outside of Greece, and its cathedral, the Agia Sofia, was the largest church in the world for a thousand years. Conquered by the Turks in 1453, Istanbul became the political centre of the Ottoman Empire. When her soldier husband set sail for Asia Minor, where he was to await battle orders for the Crimean Peninsula, Grandma Gropp followed. She stayed on the eastern shore of the Bosporus Strait in 1856, at a time when parts of Greece were still under Ottoman rule:

> I have seen a pretty great part of the world, but never found a place, which could be compared to it. The palace, we lived in, was built immitiately on the shores of the Bosporus, so that, the baywindow were I sat, was directly above the water. The Golden Horn and the Constantinopel with it's towers and minarets, was opposit me, as lying on a tray. Many big warships, and hunderd of Cayk's, sailed every day past me and by and by this little boats came under my window, offering, real mountains of splendyd cherry's and other fruit, for sale. The one side of the water, was lined with many marbel palaces, but the other side rose

softly hillward, like the Berea, only that this hills were covered with almost black looking Cipresses, through which shone the withe Villas and minarets. The latter ones had all on the top a balustade all round, which were brilliantly ligthed at night, and when allaround everything was black, this wreath's of shining light, looked, as if they were hanging in the air all round this wonderfull Oval of water.

This sojourn, in 'a little palace of the Sultan' where the officers' wives were billeted, ended along with the Crimean War. At around the time that British major John Shakespear settled on Corfu and took the historical photographs I had admired at Mon Repos, my great-great-grandparents migrated to South Africa, seduced by a dodgy deal from an unscrupulous colonial government. Therein, as Grandma Gropp would say, 'hangs an other tale.'

CHAPTER EIGHT
KEFALONIA, AND LANDFALL
ON ITHACA

THE BUS ARRIVED AT eleven o'clock on the dot, heaping scorn on my assumption that village transportation might not run to schedule. A forty-minute trip took us to the bus station in Argostoli, the capital of Kefalonia and home to around ten thousand people. The earthquakes of 1953 shook much of it to the ground, but the rebuilt town is still a pretty settlement on the banks of the Bay of Argostoli and the adjacent Koutavos Lagoon.

Along the paved lagoon-side promenade, I came to a quaintly worded sign about the twenty-seven amiable loggerheads known to frequent these waters. 'Sea turtles are peaceful animals and do not attack people,' it advised. 'But be careful, when you see a turtle, no to put your hand in the water; she might think it is food and try to bite it.'

There was also a flotilla of colourful watercraft: spindly water-bikes, small electric boats, and chunky pedalboats resembling toy cars with a hint of VW Beetle in their design. As I passed the rental stand, I couldn't help glancing back over my shoulder. At that slight sign of interest, a cheerful young man emerged from the shade of an umbrella, his T-shirt emblazoned with the words 'Argostoli Lagoon Activities Kefalonia'.

Business was slow, with only one other boat out on the lagoon, and he put his most excellent sales patter into practice, persuading me that, even though I don't drive and have never been in control of any kind of boat, not even a kayak, I was capable of managing any of his vessels for hire. Half won over, I asked which craft would be the safest. 'Not for me,' I explained, 'but for everyone else, including the turtles.' We settled on a pedalboat, a bright blue-and-white one.

It took energetic cycling to get to the middle of the lagoon, where the water lapped my boat as I oversteered and, attempting to correct my course, oversteered again. Freed from my usual inhibition, I could experiment with this new mode of transport with no one about to witness my lack of coordination.

Until an enormous loggerhead surfaced beside me.

I froze, mid-pedal. In the ripples and sunlight, she looked like a turtle-shaped pane of golden stained glass. She stayed with me for a few moments, swimming alongside the boat when I resumed pedalling. Then she veered away, and I decided not to follow, basking instead in the afterglow of the encounter.

After an hour on the water, I grew curious about the zigzag bridge separating the lagoon from the Bay of Argostoli. Back on shore, a sign claimed the De Bosset Bridge was 'the biggest stone bridge of Europe' at close to seven hundred metres in length. Instead of heading straight across the water, it has two sharp turns. The angles make it stronger and better able to withstand the waves and tides. According to the sign — which stated that the bridge is 'maybe the best link of Argostoli to the past' — the bridge's construction was the result of a fiery debate in 1812.

Charles Philippe de Bosset, an English officer of Swiss birth who became governor of the island, was struggling to convince his council to let him build the bridge:

> Then, the commander De Bosset, wrathfully pulled his sword, and placing it on the table said decisively 'My sword will solve the Gordian Knot!' In a time period of 15 days, he constructed a wooden ram bridge which connected Argostoli with the opposite coast.

The Gordian Knot, incidentally, refers to a legend reminiscent of King Arthur's sword in the stone, although it's been around a lot longer than the story of Camelot. It was said to be a knot so intricately tangled that only the next ruler of Asia would be able to unravel it. Alexander the Great, with his striking talent for getting to the heart of a problem, is said to have sliced through the elaborate tangle with one sweep of his sword. He went on to conquer a large part of Asia, extending his empire all the way from the Mediterranean Sea to India, so maybe there was something to be said for the legend. And for Alexander's direct approach to problem solving.

De Bosset was no Alexander, but he seems to have won the day. Over the next four years, they built stone arches along the bridge, and erected a marble obelisk with inscriptions glorifying Britain. Major renovations in the 1820s and 1840s enlarged, strengthened and ornamented the bridge. The first cars drove across in the 1920s, but it is now reserved for pedestrians.

War and natural disaster have taken their toll:

> At 1940 the Italian bombardments caused cracks on the bridge. The years of Italian occupation of the island (1941–1943) the conquerors erased the phrases written on the obelisk. At 1944, the Germans placed explosive devices along the waterfront and the bridge of Argostoli... They intended to set off the explosives while leaving the island, in September of the same year. Fortunately,

local soldiers, co-operating with Italian and Slovenian soldiers, cut the wires and saved the bridge and the city. The big earthquake of February 1867 caused important damages on the bridge and the obelisk. Though, bigger damage was caused by the disastrous earthquake of 1953.

I paced across the bridge and back again, pausing to examine the obelisk and two keen fishers: on one side of the bridge was a cormorant perched on a timber post jutting out of the lagoon, its eyes fixed on a point below the surface; on the other, a grizzled old man stood thigh-deep in the shallows, pulling his day's catch from the bay with a handheld net.

There was just enough time to visit the ornate Church of Theotokos Sissiotissa, from where, the same sign informed me, the Holy Cross is taken to the bridge and 'thrown into the water'. Assuming this was an enthusiastic mistranslation, I looked it up online. A bit of internet browsing indicated that the ceremony might be a little more restrained, with the congregation taking the cross to the bridge each year on the feast of the Epiphany and dipping it into the bay. But, when I read a story in Victoria Hislop's *Cartes Postales from Greece*, in which youths competed to recover a cross flung into the sea by a Greek Orthodox priest, I wasn't so sure. Much later, at one of our book club gatherings back in Australia, I asked Kate to find out more about the ritual from her island contacts. She checked with a Kefalonian school headmistress, who told her, 'It goes into the water, but swimmers dive in and retrieve it.'

The last bus back to Svoronata left at 1.40 p.m., so I had only two hours for this interlude in Argostoli, and I relished every minute. A timetable at the central bus station confirmed there was no public transport from the village on weekends, so it was just as well I'd signed up for tours on both days.

~ ~ ~

Saturday's excursion promised to tick two of my boxes: Ithaca and Fiskardo. It was advertised, rather ambitiously, as a 'Venetian Voyage', though I suspected the only thing Venetian about it would be Fiskardo's architecture.

The early bus wound its way around the route to Argostoli, picking up passengers from one hotel after another. At last, it reached the island's capital and curved around the lagoon where I'd pedalled with such exultant energy the day before. From there, we'd drive across the island to its eastern coast, where our boat would be waiting. Before we headed inland, though, our coach had to drive along a nerve-wracking cliff.

My window seat was on the side of the bus away from the precipice. The road was narrow, the curves blind, and there were times we slowed to edge past oncoming cars, but at least I didn't have to stare into the abyss. Unfortunately, I couldn't help but overhear the running commentary from the man next to me. Leaning across the aisle to his wife and daughter, he was gleefully pointing out the various places where rockfalls or wayward vehicles had dented or crashed through the flimsy roadside barrier.

Even before our juddering halt to avoid colliding with an oncoming truck, I was way outside my comfort zone. But I could hardly ask the driver to stop and let me off. All I could do was memorise the locations of the emergency exits. I already had my eye on the little red hammer I'd use to bash out my window and escape from a watery grave.

When we arrived at the harbour of Agia Efimia, we swapped our perilous bus for a much more reassuring boat.

The boat's first stop was in a cove off the island of Ithaca. This, more than anywhere else I'd yet visited, was a direct connection with the tales of antiquity. Ithaca may well have been the realm of Odysseus the Cunning, the mastermind behind the wooden Trojan Horse that brought about Troy's defeat after a decade-long war. It took another ten years of misadventure for him to get home, as Homer tells it in *The Odyssey*. When he at last reached his kingdom of Ithaca, disguised as a beggar, no one recognised him. No one, that is, except for his dog, as it lay on a dung heap dying of age and neglect. It's hard to forgive Odysseus for letting this loyal friend die alone without a single comforting pat, even though that might have blown his cover. Come to think of it, it's hard to forgive him his atrocities both at war and at home, even if they weren't considered crimes in his day. But I was still smitten with the idea of treading the same earth he once trod.

I was one of the first from our boat to plunge into the cool waters off Ithaca. The sea glittered where it reflected the sunshine, but was wine-dark in the shadow of the hills that rose from the shore. Their slopes, blanketed in thick bushes and trees, looked to be impenetrable, despite the occasional house peeking out from the vegetation. This rugged landscape, some archaeologists believe, is the most likely site of Odysseus's settlement.

Unlike my fellow day-trippers, who were splashing around close to the boat, I swam to shore. I wanted to plant my feet on Ithaca, but it was too painful to walk onto the stony beach, so I sat down and scooted back on my bum until I got to dry land. My feet stayed in the water, but I successfully planted my bottom on Odysseus's island.

Refreshed from the swim, we cruised on to the village of Fiskardo near the northern tip of Kefalonia. Fiskardo's claim to fame is that it still showcases buildings constructed through the centuries, even though the 1953 earthquakes levelled most of the island. It is a charming harbourside town that has become a tourist drawcard.

Our guide warned us to use our free time wisely by choosing a place for lunch right away. We were the first tourist boat to dock that day, but she warned us that larger craft would arrive soon, and it might become difficult to get a table.

I wandered past various restaurants along the waterfront until I reached Tselenti. Built by the current owner's grandfather as a summer residence in the late nineteenth century, it had served as a school and a wartime police station before becoming Fiskardo's first hotel in 1967. Here, I indulged in the most delectable meal of the trip, with a price tag to match: expensive for Greece, but not unreasonable in Australian dollars.

I started with a mojito. With all that mint and lime, after all, it's practically a salad. Then, as I soaked in the outdoor café vibe, I chose a couple of appetisers and a dessert, instead of a main course. After spiced feta in delicate filo pastry drizzled with honey and sesame seeds, and an array of roasted Mediterranean vegetables, I finished up with a slice of strawberry cheesecake covered in coulis and cream.

There was more than an hour until the boat was due to leave, so I sought out the old Roman cemetery and then returned to browse the harbourside boutiques. Shopping soon bored me, until I came across a map showing three walking tracks. By far the shortest, the Lighthouse Trail would take half an hour and end near the dock where our boat waited. A glance at my wrist confirmed there were still forty minutes until our departure, so I set off along the rocky woodland path. For a fleeting, no doubt mojito-enhanced moment, I looked up and saw dozens of tiny blue-and-white pennants fluttering in the trees. It took a second for my gaze to focus. There were no flags, just glimpses of the sapphire sky revealed by the trembling dance of sun-blanched leaves.

An uphill hike took me to the ruins of a Byzantine basilica. Early Christians began building this church in the sixth century, and it is one of the oldest on the Ionian islands. Through its crumbling, keyhole-shaped doors and windows, it offered views of greenery stretching to hazy mountains on the horizon.

Following timber signs along the trail, I found my way to two lighthouses: the obelisk-like tower of the 'new' lighthouse, built in 1892, and the much shorter round tower of the sixteenth-century Venetian lighthouse, a chess piece against the bright skies. The day was hot, but the walls of the older lighthouse were cool to the touch, as were the succulent, graffiti-scarred leaves of a nearby cactus. Surprisingly, the Venetian tower's door stood open, so I climbed its thirty-three spiral steps — with great caution, as the lunchtime cocktail had left me a teensy bit tipsy.

After a glorious ocean swim in glossy waters off another deserted beach, our boat took us back to Agia Efimia. Throughout the day, I'd been dreading the return bus trip, this time in the outside lane. Although it was a different vehicle, we all sat in the same arrangement as we had that morning. As one does. When I dropped into my seat, the first thing I did was give my seatbelt a gentle tug, pulling it towards me so I could buckle in.

The entire mechanism came loose and landed in my lap.

I placed the broken belt discreetly under the seat and took a deep breath, determined to appreciate the view. It was an impressive one, with olive trees growing almost horizontally out of the steep gradient from the road to the sea below. *Good*, I thought, gazing down at them. *If we go off the road, we won't plummet all the way into the water. At least the trees will slow our crashing fall. But what is it with me and buses? Are they out to get me?*

I'd been congratulating myself on overcoming my fear but, as my muscles tensed with anxiety, the long-ago accident in Sri Lanka didn't seem so far away. Silent echoes of that collision disturbed the air trapped inside our bus, inaudible to the cheerful day-trippers chatting around me.

CHAPTER NINE
MEMORIES OF SRI LANKA

Silence, broken by children's cries.

A gradual awareness of fluid running down my neck.

An unhurried examination of the redness coating my fingertips and the intriguing thought, It's blood. *And then:* It's my blood.

The clump of fair hair, torn from someone's scalp, lying at my feet. I considered it with careful logic until I worked out from the colour that it must be mine.

THIRTEEN MONTHS AFTER THE 2004 Boxing Day tsunami devastated south-east Asia and shocked the world, I travelled to the island nation of Sri Lanka.

At the time of the natural disaster, I was a primary school teacher in the United Arab Emirates and had been planning a holiday in Sri Lanka with Pierre, my then-boyfriend. I was at a clinic getting travel vaccinations when I first saw footage of the tsunami's dreadful aftermath. Against the background of so much suffering, tourism seemed disrespectful, and we put our trip on hold.

One of the kids in my class was Sri Lankan, and her mother, Nirupa, travelled home to help. Nirupa's mission was to supply sanitary towels to women who had lost everything, helping them maintain their dignity when life had dealt them such a cruel blow. International aid organisations were distributing food, shelter and essential medical treatment but, as so often happens, this basic female need was in danger of being overlooked. Through her fundraising, I felt a connection to a country facing massive adversity, including a shattered tourism industry. So, when picking a holiday destination a year later, I knew it was important to revive our plans. Pierre wasn't comfortable visiting a place so vulnerable to disaster, so I travelled alone.

That solo journey through Sri Lanka was a festival of the senses. I marvelled at the sight of a colossal reclining Buddha carved into living rock, squeezed water from my drenched hair after a monsoon downpour, inhaled the scent of Ayurvedic herbs as I lay in a wooden box to steam the fatigue from my travel-weary limbs. In Kandy, I caught my breath as dancers leapt into the air, their bright orange sarongs lifting and swirling around them. At Pinnawala Elephant Orphanage, I laughed with joy as a rescued baby elephant tugged at the bottle of milk in my hands, then watched in sadness as a three-legged adult — the victim of a landmine — limped down to the river to bathe.

An ascent between massive stone lion's paws took me to the plateau atop the fortress rock of Sigiriya. There I stood, as if on an island, looking down at an ocean of treetops 180 metres below. At nearby Dambulla, a neat, white temple façade gazed out from under a brooding brow of rock. Inside its five caves, the air was cool and more than 150 statues of the Buddha lined the painted walls.

A train ticket to the hill country of the southern interior cost the rupee equivalent of one Australian dollar and change, and it took me on a four-hour, seventy-kilometre journey into the heart of the tea plantation region. My eyes feasted on the rolling green landscape — so different from the arid flatness of Abu Dhabi — and my ears danced to the drumming of a friendly jam session echoing the *clack-clack* of the train.

With no available seats, I was one of those who sat for a while in an open doorway, my back resting against the steel plate of the carriage wall, and my left arm hooked around a metal bar. Those were the days when I still trusted in the strength of that arm.

My goal was to summit Sri Pada, also known as Adam's Peak. Turning down the opportunity of hiring a car and driver, I travelled on a series of local buses: from the town of Nuwara Eliya to the village of Hatton; from Hatton to the hamlet of Maskeliya; from Maskeliya to the base of the mountain. This last vehicle, a minibus designed to hold eighteen people, transported the driver, twenty-one seated passengers and at least ten standing, most of us clutching bulky bags of belongings.

An ancient pilgrimage route leads to the top of Sri Pada, 2,243 metres above sea level. Here, some believe, the Buddha left his footprint in the rock on his final visit to Sri Lanka. Others claim it was the Biblical Adam's foot that made its mark when he arrived on Earth. Still others believe the indentation to be the footprint of the Hindu Lord Shiva. Something about this place has inspired the followers of many different faiths.

My *Lonely Planet* advised a two o'clock start to catch the sunrise, so I dragged myself from my hostel bed at that ghastly hour and began a breathless climb up 5,200 steps in the chilly darkness. Struggling upward, I crossed paths with Sri Lankans descending from their own pilgrimages. A surprising number were elderly women, barefoot and seemingly unperturbed by the physical demands of the track.

I reached the mountaintop temple around 5.30 a.m., an hour before daybreak. Scores of Sri Lankans and a couple of dozen tourists huddled and shivered together on the steps outside the gate to the sacred enclosure. As the sun appeared above the horizon, silence descended on pilgrims and travellers alike, awestruck by the majestic view illuminated in the dawn light. Buddhist monks in warm knitted beanies, coloured saffron to match their robes, emerged to prepare the day's offerings.

~ ~ ~

On 27 January 2006, I was the only foreigner on a crowded bus, revelling in the adventure of finding my way from one place to another. My eyes were on the pages of the guidebook in my lap when we overtook a truck and slammed into another bus, which was doing the same thing in the opposite direction.

My overriding impression of Sri Lanka is neither the beauty of its holy sites nor the trauma of the accident. It is the utter kindness of its people.

The driver and passengers of a third bus interrupted their daily lives to carry the injured to the nearest town. In a region scarred by poverty, these passersby took the trouble to leave my bags at a police station. I lost only two possessions: my glasses, ripped from my face on impact, and the close-fitting T-shirt that I begged the nurses to cut from my torso rather than tug over my tortured neck and head. I was shrieking with pain by the time they brought out the scissors, to a chorus of disapproving grumbles at the wastefulness of destroying a near-new garment.

Staff from Gajaba, the small hotel where I'd stayed the night before, arrived soon after I came out of surgery to reassure me that I was not alone. I later discovered they had brought sheets and pillows. These were luxury items, not supplied by the hospital. Most of the other patients had relatives camping out on the floor beside their beds, providing their linen, food and basic nursing care.

The Samaritans I can never thank enough, though, were two contacts Nirupa had given me before I left Abu Dhabi. One was Aruna, the father of a little boy in our school, whose family she'd arranged for me to visit in Kandy. The other was Chamila, Nirupa's sister in Colombo. 'In case you need something,' she said.

Aruna heard about the accident on the radio moments before I called. The anaesthetist had sought me out and volunteered his personal mobile phone, dialling the numbers for me as I lay on a gurney in a busy corridor — it was a six-hour wait for an operation to remove glass from my body and put a total of thirty-eight stitches in my neck, forehead, knee and one unlucky finger. As far as I could make out, the hospital itself had no working telephone.

At the kind-hearted anaesthetist's urging, I made a second call, to Pierre in Abu Dhabi. My memory of these conversations is blurred: I remember nothing of the first and, of the second, only the note of ragged helplessness in Pierre's voice. The calls were just in case things went wrong, so my family could find out what had happened. I didn't expect anyone to *do* anything. And there was nothing Pierre could do. But Aruna left his home long before sunrise and travelled for three hours over unlit, potholed jungle roads to reach me by half past six on the morning after the accident.

He brought tender morsels of fruit his wife had prepared to tempt an unwilling appetite, and gently fed me the few mouthfuls he could coax me to eat. He tracked down my belongings, dealt with the police and insurance company, found a neck brace — goodness knows where, since the medical staff hadn't given me one. He phoned around the world to notify my friends and family, dealing with their shock and queries.

And he struggled to have me discharged. Polonnaruwa's hospital was rudimentary; it has since been transformed and supplemented by a glossy new facility, but I recognise the run-down clinic in the pages of Michael Ondaatje's *Anil's Ghost*. Aruna was determined to move me to Apollo Hospital, one of the finest medical facilities in Sri Lanka's capital city.

Aruna knew that waiting for an ambulance to drive from Colombo would add excruciating hours to my distress, and dangerous ones, too, if my neck injury turned out to be serious. He negotiated with police, doctors, and a reluctant insurance company until they allowed him to take me on the five-hour journey himself. He hired a vehicle and driver so he could sit in the back seat, letting me grip his hand when the pain overwhelmed me. When necessary, this quiet, reserved man helped me get to a toilet. He stood just outside the door, so he could hear if I called out or fell to the ground.

In Colombo, where he'd arranged for a representative from my travel insurance company to meet us at the hospital, Aruna made sure I was safely in her care before setting off with a flat phone battery on the long road to Kandy. It would have been well after midnight before he reached his wife and young children.

Nirupa's sister Chamila and her family arrived at Apollo Hospital shortly after I did and stayed with me through the ordeal of MRIs, CAT scans and X-rays. They left around midnight and were back the next morning. She repeatedly made the six-hour round trip, brought me new clothes and took my blood-soaked garments home to wash. In fact, she took all my laundry, and I was mortified that she was dealing with the smelly, travel-stained clothing in which I had traipsed, hiked and climbed through humid cities and countryside. Chamila invited me to stay in her home if I needed somewhere to go when the hospital discharged me. She was willing to take care of me, knowing I would require help with even the most distasteful bodily functions.

~ ~ ~

Once installed in a private room, I could have been in any modern hospital anywhere in the world. This room, along with a narrow glimpse of the hallway whenever the door slid open, became my world for the next week and a half.

For long days and nights, I lay flat on my back, the slightest movement of my torso driving shafts of pain through my neck. I had lost a lot of blood but had been adamant, going into surgery, that I didn't want a transfusion, given the potential health risks involved. This left me weak and, after the first, worst few days, voraciously hungry.

Three times a day, a meal was placed on a tray over my bed. I could reach up to feed myself, but I couldn't see the food. Identifying dishes by touch and the taste on my fingertips after I dipped them into unseen bowls, I found soups and dahl curries and tasty sauces that were just about impossible to eat from my horizontal position. Sometimes a bowl of jelly was the most solid item on the menu. At least I could scoop it up with my fingers and carry it to my lips with a minimum of mess.

The doctors seemed concerned at what they presumed was my lack of appetite, but it took a couple of days for me to pluck up the nerve to ask if I could have a sandwich for lunch. Its midday arrival became the pivot around which each slow day turned.

Oh, how I longed for lunchtime and its simple sandwich — always cheese and tomato on slices of white bread as soft and insubstantial as the mists that clung to Sri Pada. I'd chew it with careful relish, but it would sate my hunger for barely an hour before the craving returned. Meanwhile, my flesh melted away. In the weeks after I left the hospital, I more than made up for this, satisfying prodigious hankerings for food, especially the red meat that had been absent from the hospital fare, and gaining a weight problem that has stayed with me to this day.

Even here, in this high-tech hospital with its sandwiches and private rooms, I continued to experience remarkable kindness.

There was a student nurse whom I remember well. Her name was Ayesha, and she would make time to help with my morning or evening meal, spoon-feeding me dishes I had to leave uneaten on her days off.

Roshanee, the travel insurance rep, comforted me when my spirits were low. The hours stretched from one dose of pain medication to the next, and by her second visit, I was desperate for something to read. When she brought me a book, it was disturbing to find my mind skittering, unable to concentrate. For the first time in my life, I was incapable of losing myself in the words on a page.

My room had a television set high on the wall opposite the bed but, without my glasses, its flickering light brought on throbbing headaches. The TV was a blessing, though. Word soon got out that I wasn't averse to company, despite the language barrier. At intervals, there would be a quiet tap on the door. If I called out a greeting, it would open to reveal a hospital orderly or janitor. I'd fumble for the remote control lying close to hand and click the TV on to the international cricket test series between Sri Lanka, South Africa and Australia. There'd soon be up to five silent young men lined up in the narrow space between the bed and the wall, catching a few stolen minutes of the game until another knock on the door signalled the approach of a supervisor, I guessed, and they'd fade away.

A woman who worked as a nanny and cleaner in the home of one of my Emirati pupils was in Colombo at that time, visiting her family. Months later, I discovered that she'd used scarce resources on a two-hour commute to the hospital, only to be turned away because she didn't know my surname.

There was one exception to the otherwise universal kindness I experienced in Sri Lanka.

One of the things good nurses do is wean patients away from physical dependency. Several days into my hospital stay, a nurse helped me into my little bathroom, propped me up against the handbasin, and insisted I brush my teeth unaided while she watched from the doorway, just short steps away. I tried to warn her when my mind dissolved in a fizzy rush, but the words slithered away from me, and she couldn't get to me before I lost consciousness, jarring my whiplashed neck as my body smacked into the floor. Put straight to bed, I lay motionless in miserable pain. Every small gain I had made in the preceding days, every inch of recovery, had been lost.

It was during this lowest point that someone entered the room and rifled through my bedside cabinet. I could hear what was happening, but I couldn't even open my eyes as I listened to somebody steal the only diamond I've ever owned: a tiny chip of a thing in a setting I'd had custom designed, bought with the paycheque from my first professional job. It was far too frivolous an item to replace, and not worth whinging about in the greater scheme of things, but that little gemstone had meant something to me.

I suspect I know who the culprit was — someone not mentioned in these pages, by name or otherwise.

~ ~ ~

I spent three weeks in Sri Lanka: seven days exploring, twelve in its hospitals, and another three in a hotel room before the doctors cleared me to fly home with a professional nurse escort.

My sister Tassin, herself a qualified nurse, also flew from Australia to be with me. She arranged for my discharge from hospital to a nearby hotel until I was well enough to fly. There, she sat me in the shower so she could wash the last of the blood out of my hair. I needed her care, as I was unable to get up by myself. At most, she could help me into a wheelchair for short periods of time before the pain and fatigue drove me to my bed. Holding my head up with the brace on was exhausting; without its support, the effort was agonising.

I had a taste of how society sidelines people who use wheelchairs when a porter parked me in a corner, with my back to the room, while Tassin checked us in to the hotel. He left me isolated and vulnerable, staring at the walls that met in front of my burning face. Because of my injury, I couldn't turn my head even a fraction of an inch. The depth of my humiliation stunned me.

Worse still was after our plane landed in Abu Dhabi. While everyone else exited down the steps on the left, an airline official wheeled me to the right where an open door gaped high above the ground. When he reversed onto the mechanised platform that had been raised to receive me, there was a sharp jolt as the wheelchair dropped a centimetre or three from plane to platform. Unwarned, I felt the terror of falling from a great height, followed a microsecond later by the pain of impact.

My other memory of this flight — my first and only taste of long-haul business class, paid for by the insurance company as a medical evacuation — was my nurse giving the okay for a single glass of champagne. I managed a couple of clumsy sips, but the precious liquid was spilling down my neck, so I ended up sipping through a straw, with Tassin tilting the glass for me to reach the last drops.

My family had ignored my assurances that I could cope on my own, and I am so thankful they did. Tassin's mercy trip led, indirectly, to my immigration to Australia and to meeting Adam. Years later, Aruna and his family visited Australia and we had a chance to host them overnight at Walkabout Park, Tassin's animal sanctuary. The children had grown, and it was a delight to take them behind the scenes so they could interact with the animals and choose keepsakes from the gift shop. Nothing we could say or do, though, could measure up to our gratitude. We will never forget that, when I was a broken body on a faraway island, there was someone by my side.

While researching this chapter, I found a lengthy email that Jenny wrote to Aruna twelve days after the accident:

> Good morning, Aruna, from a cold and rainy Johannesburg in South Africa.
>
> My name is Jenny, and I am Sally's older sister.
>
> I needed to contact you to try and convey to you how much you mean to Sally, myself, and all the rest of her friends and family.
>
> On the 28th, as soon as you had spoken to Sally's friend Megan in Cape Town, she called me to tell me that Sally had been involved in a terrible bus accident in Sri Lanka, and that she was being moved to Colombo because her neck was badly injured.

At that point, we did not understand that you were with her as her friend and companion, and we were very upset that she was facing this trouble in her life all on her own.

So, on the 22nd, our other sister, Tassin, who lives in Sydney, Australia called me, and we decided that one of us (or maybe both of us) should travel to Sri Lanka to be with her. We then found out the details of what you had done for Sally — how you travelled through the night to be with her, dealt with the first hospital, the police, and the insurance company, how you transported her safely to Colombo, and then stayed with her until she was safely in the hospital. We also realised that you had organised very strong support for her, from other people as well.

You must be a wonderful man to do everything that you did for her — even though she was nearly a stranger to you. I know that you are probably aware of what you did for her — but I don't think that you understand that everything you did was not just for Sally, but also for all of us who know and love her.

All around the world, Sally's friends and family could deal with her situation better, because we knew that you were close to her, and had helped her when she was unable to help herself.

Tassin arrived in Sri Lanka last night. This morning, Sally was discharged from the hospital, and she will stay in a hotel with Tassin near to the hospital, until they fly back to UAE on the 10th of February. The insurance people want her to stay near to the hospital in case there are further problems.

I cannot put into words how we feel. So many times when we talk about what has happened to her, we say to each other: 'How do you thank someone like Aruna?' We feel that there is nothing that we can do or say to make you fully realise how grateful we are to you.

When she was in the hospital, I asked her to write down the story of what had happened to her. She said that she did not want to, as it is such a terrible story. I then said to her that this is not a terrible story — it is a story of beauty, as we have all learned that there are still wonderful people in a world that sometimes feels very cruel. And you are the main reason that we have new faith in the goodness of people.

If you or your family should ever decide to visit South Africa or Australia, we would be honoured to welcome you into our homes, and to show you some of the kindness that you have shown Sally — although I don't think that we can ever fully repay you.

So I ask you to please accept our deepest thanks, and know that you have a very special place in many, many hearts.

Jenny

CHAPTER TEN
KICKING BACK ON
KEFALONIA

I T HAD BEEN MORE than a decade since that Sri Lankan misadventure, but in some ways it would always be with me. The bus ride along the coastal cliffs of Kefalonia passed as a series of sphincter-clenching pangs of fear. But I survived the trip back to Svoronata, relieved that my fellow passengers seemed oblivious to my distress. Suffused with gratitude and the afterglow of having challenged my demons, I invited my hosts out for a meal.

Paul drove us high into the hills to a restaurant called Il Borgo. A short pre-dinner stroll took us to Agios Georgios Kastro, a sixteenth-century Venetian castle that served as the capital of Kefalonia for two centuries. Then, over a meaty casserole and a shared bottle of wine, I told them about my day. My words effervesced with the high of having made landfall on Odysseus's island, so it was a bit deflating when Paul, who was born on Kefalonia, explained that the siting of the legendary kingdom on the island known today as Ithaca is only theoretical. As we sipped glasses of *mastika*, a resin-flavoured liqueur that slipped down my throat like polished fire, he put forward an alternative hypothesis: that the Ithaca of the Bronze Age was located on one of Kefalonia's peninsulas, with the larger island having changed its shape in the geological upheavals of the intervening millennia.

~ ~ ~

Sunday's expedition was billed as one of discovery, and the first thing I discovered when re-reading the blurb was that our lunch stop would be in Agia Efimia, the same harbourside village from which our boat had sailed the day before. This meant I'd have to brave at least one more bus journey along the same terrifying road. I wasn't keen on the idea, but I resolved I could do it.

Our first stop was at the monastery of Saint Gerasimos, where the relics of the island's patron saint, venerated as a healer, rest in a silver-and-glass casket. The saint is said to wander the night in times of tribulation, bringing comfort to those in need, and his miracles make for a memorable scene in *Captain Corelli's Mandolin*.

The monastery is an important religious centre, so I had taken care to dress appropriately. My Greek goddess dress, purchased in Athens the previous year, had a long skirt, and the shawl swathed around my shoulders covered my upper arms and any trace of cleavage. Nevertheless, despite the best of intentions, I behaved shamefully.

Our guide assured us that, even though the Sunday morning service was in progress, the congregation welcomed visitors. I'm not sure why it didn't occur to me that this was a questionable assertion.

We filed off the bus and into the church's vestibule. Like many others from our coach, I slotted a few coins into the collection box and lit a candle. The rest of the group soon left to mill around the courtyard, but I made my quiet way further inside and found a single vacant seat. An elaborate sarcophagus lay across the crowded nave, though the body of the saint within was not visible. I kept my head bowed and eyes lowered in deference to the Greek Orthodox worshippers all around.

A grandmother's brusque stilling of a fidgeting child gave me an inward smile as I remembered my own Roman Catholic upbringing, and that time my mother yanked me back by the collar when I forgot to genuflect before entering a pew. I savoured this slight connection with the people around me, even though I didn't share their faith. I sat when the congregation sat and stood when they stood, staying as long as I could before I needed to rejoin the coach.

Just as I rose to leave, the service reached its most sacred moments. Everyone knelt, many with their knees pressed into the hard floors of the aisles, and the church that had seemed crowded when I'd arrived was now absolutely packed with wall-to-wall praying bodies.

The choice in front of me was a poor one. If I didn't leave immediately, I'd delay a coachload of sightseers. I had already stepped away from my seat and was standing in the aisle, a blemish among the pious parishioners, so I picked my way through the kneeling worshippers with care. My clumsiness hampered me, though, and my whispered apologies disturbed the devotions around me. I left in disgrace, aware that I should have been far more mindful before intruding on the prayers of the faithful.

Our tour moved on to a winery where I bought a couple of bottles of the island's dry white Robola, sewn into hessian covers in a nod to the sacks once used to protect cartloads of bottles on rough trails. The winery didn't sell corkscrews, missing out on a sure source of income. Fortunately, there was a tacky 'I love Kefalonia' corkscrew for sale at our next stop, Drogarati Cave, where we descended into the earth to admire its dramatic stalactites and stalagmites. It was my dad who'd taught us kids the difference between the two. 'When the mites run up,' he used to laugh, 'the tights come down.' We'd giggle and squirm at the idea of little creatures swarming inside our stockings.

Melissani was the highlight of the day, the reason I'd signed up for this tour in the first place. It is a spectacular natural pool inside a cave, reached via a pedestrian ramp that tunnels through the rock. The light at the end of this tunnel is a vertical sunbeam striking the lake, a result of the cave roof collapsing in times long past to reveal the sky. The mineral-rich water transforms from deep indigo to bright turquoise as it reflects the sunlight, its sparkling ripples impossible to capture with a cheap phone camera.

The lake is fed from an underground stream that flows all the way from Katavothres, the site of an old watermill on the island's west coast. It continues its subterranean travels a little further beyond Melissani to emerge in the Bay of Sami in the east, across the sea from Ithaca.

We were lucky to be able to head straight down the tunnel and, without delay, into waiting boats. The short ride took us around both the open and covered parts of the cave, where our coxswain sang to us in the dark as his oars lapped the water. When we got back to dry land, we had to shuffle past scores of tourists queueing for their turn.

On the way out, I stopped in the souvenir shop to buy a gold-coloured headband of fake laurel leaves. Paired with the dress I was wearing, this would be the basis of my costume for the next Australian Discworld Convention, a biennial gathering of fellow Terry Pratchett aficionados. It would be my fifth convention, but the first where I would cosplay it up with my geeky friends. I would be playing a minor character in Pratchett's books: Anoia, the goddess of things that get stuck in drawers. A belt hung with ladles and potato mashers, together with a shawl sewn with smaller kitchen utensils, would complete the outfit.

At our lunch stop, I logged into the restaurant's Wi-Fi. While tucking into a Kefalonian meat pie — a local speciality of filo pastry filled with beef, goat and pork mixed with rice — I checked WhatsApp to find out how my brother was doing in South Africa. While I was toasting my middlescent life in a taverna overlooking the harbour, he was celebrating his by running the Comrades Ultra-Marathon.

Our sister Jenny had flown from Johannesburg to Durban to support Michael by watching him run through a series of checkpoints. I felt I was doing my bit simply by being in Greece, the home of the legendary marathon of ancient times.

The Battle of Marathon took place in 490 BCE, during one of Persia's attempts to invade Greece. Herodotus, who was born six years after this campaign, wrote that the Athenians sent a man named Pheidippides to the Peloponnese Peninsula. His urgent mission was to summon Sparta's warriors to help repel the Persians. Pheidippides ran the entire way, 221 kilometres as Google Maps flies, only for the Spartans to turn him down. They were observing a religious festival and could not, by their law, march to the aid of Athens until the moon was full. What could Pheidippides do, but run home with the bad news?

My *tetarto* of wine — a quarter kilo, or 250 millilitres, because house wines are commonly ordered by weight in Greece — arrived as I was pondering how long it had taken the bus to drive from Athens to Sparta during my first Greek trip. *At least Pheidippides wouldn't have had to cross the vertigo-inducing chasm that is now the Corinth Canal*, I thought, remembering how I'd retreated after only a few steps onto the walkway that shuddered and shook with each heavy vehicle passing over the bridge.

A later but better-known version of the story claims Pheidippides ran from Marathon to Athens, a much more manageable forty kilometres. He delivered the news of the Greeks' victory in battle before collapsing in an exhausted heap and dying on the spot. It is said that he gasped out the word '*Niki*' with his last breath, referring to the goddess of victory and the triumph she brought to the Greeks. I wonder how many Nike-shod athletes today realise, as they line up to begin their own marathons, that every pounding step will be a tribute to the winged goddess of old.

In honour of this legend, the marathon race was inaugurated at the first modern international Olympics, held in Athens in 1896. In a wise move, the organisers went with the later tale and its shorter, forty-kilometre track.

The standard distance for a marathon has since been set as 42.195 kilometres, based on the route at the 1908 London Summer Olympics. Why the extra two-and-a-bit, you might ask? Some say it was on a royal whim, with Princess Mary wanting the race to start outside the windows of the palace nursery, so her children could witness the event.

My brother was running an ultra-marathon, which is more than twice as long as the regular race. The route measured eighty-nine gruelling kilometres. Jenny was following his progress and keeping the rest of us siblings — Tassin, Andrew, Brian and me — posted on WhatsApp. By the time I logged in, she'd watched him pass Kilometre 7 and Kilometre 33, but had missed him at Kilometre 50. She had an app that told her he'd gone through, so she drove to the next checkpoint in the hope she would see him there.

An anxious message popped up on the screen while I ate: 'His running partner has gone through a checkpoint without him.'

I lost contact when I got on the coach but, as soon as I arrived home, I checked in again. Michael, despite slowing down considerably, had finished the race: 'All good but the reason for the problem in the middle is that his chest closed so they are giving him a bit of nebulising before we take him home.'

He spent the evening in the local hospital before medical personnel cleared him to fly. In addition to those given trackside aid, Jenny told us, the hospital treated around eight hundred runners that day. Seventeen were triaged as 'Code Red'. This means that about one in every thousand people who attempted the ultra-marathon ended up with life-threatening disorders. Just like Pheidippides.

When I asked Michael if it was an asthma attack — we'd spent many days wheezing in adjacent twin beds as children — he replied, 'Yip. It felt different. Rather than being a feeling of "lungs not expanding enough" it was a sudden "collapsing of my throat" and the air just couldn't get through.' Nevertheless, his smartwatch registered 102,018 steps, making my own daily Fitbit counts look pathetic by comparison.

~ ~ ~

No longer worried about Michael, I unpacked the care package Linda had left at my door. It contained artichoke stew for my dinner, cinnamon-dusted rice pudding for tomorrow's breakfast, and a last small load of clean clothes, neatly folded. Tucked in the side of the laundry basket was an impressive book of artworks created by Paul's brother, Yerassimos Sklavos, some of whose sculptures I'd seen dotted around the island.

As I flipped through its pages, I considered the weekend's group tourism experiences. On Saturday, it had felt as if I were travelling on my own, just happening to share a means of transportation with a bunch of strangers. There was little tourist commentary and no group activity, just a gentle boat trip with two invigorating swimming breaks and a visit to Fiskardo, where I enjoyed a solo lunch and a memorable short hike. Sunday's tour, though, had been a little tacky, with the guide herding us from place to place. The coach had taken us to four interesting sites I'd otherwise have missed, but the day had been more meaningful for the books I was reading than for the sightseeing I'd done.

As I closed the cover on *Captain Corelli's Mandolin*, the skilfully crafted narrative lingered in my mind. I'd read it twice before, but I hadn't known much about Greece at the time. With everything I'd learned over the last year — understanding a few Greek phrases, knowing a little about the country's history, having a feel for the landscape, being familiar with way too much of the food — I got far more out of it this time around. Plus, the emotional experience of reading it here, on Kefalonia itself, was compelling. The tale has always been a heartrending one, but now I focused on aspects that hadn't meant much to me before. The earthquake was a terrifying natural disaster that shook the book's pages, and the soldiers' voices rang in the air as they sang for the very last time.

There was a crushing poignancy in visiting the settings of the story's events. The tense scene when an armoured car appeared on the same crooked bridge I'd crossed on Friday was just one of the connections that illustrated why pairing books with places is such a rewarding pastime. Instead of simply picturing the scene in my mind's eye, I could *feel* it. I knew the breeze that ruffled the water of the bay on one side of the bridge, but merely rippled the surface of the lagoon on the other. I heard my footsteps on the paving, felt my body turn as I moved from one zigzag angle to the next, saw how a combat vehicle would dominate the narrow walkway, leaving room for no one in its path.

I surprised myself with my next e-reader download, an 1898 translation of a classic written in the eighth century BCE. It didn't take long before I got to this passage about Odysseus, who was known in Latin as Ulysses:

> Ulysses led the brave Cephallenians, who held Ithaca, Neritum with its forests, Crocylea, rugged Aegilips, Samos and Zacynthus, with the mainland also that was over against the islands. These were led by Ulysses, peer of Jove in counsel, and with him there came twelve ships.

True to form, I reached for my phone and posted a screenshot to Facebook:

4 June 2017
Paul's explanation of why the island today called Ithaca may not have been the seat of Odysseus's power has inspired me, for the first time, to tackle

Homer's *The Iliad*. Found this in Samuel Butler's translation, supporting my host's argument that the Ithaca of legend included the whole of present-day Kefalonia and more. Paul explained how the peninsula where Lixouri is now located was probably once an island and is a plausible site for Odysseus's home. I have planted neither feet nor any other part of my body on Lixouri, although I did see it from across the channel. Next time.

If I had made this discovery a year before, I might have descended through a spiralling fear of missing out, second-guessing the value of my Ithacan interlude and trying to force in a visit to Lixouri before I left Kefalonia. Now, I was content to have struck out for that pebble beach on the modern-day island of Ithaca, dreaming of Odysseus and making a memory I'd treasure forever.

CHAPTER ELEVEN
KEFALONIA TO NAFPLIO

BEFORE THEY DROPPED ME off at the airport for my flight to the mainland, my Kefalonian hosts took me to see Katavothres, the inlet of the waters that flowed deep under the island to Melissani Cave Lake and beyond. On the way, Paul stopped the car at the location of the awful climax of *Captain Corelli's Mandolin*, but we had to pull away when another vehicle sped up behind us. It was too brief a pause for me to get a sense of the place. When I'd first read this book, I assumed it was unadulterated fiction. Back in 1999, I didn't even know that Kefalonia was a real place. Now, I realised how much of the novel, even down to the arias sung in its most intense passages, was grounded in fact.

The day was long and tiring, as all days that include air travel seem to be, and I was glad I'd decided to stop over in Athens for a night's rest before continuing to Nafplio. As I checked into the Art Gallery Hotel for the last time, I remarked that Arti the cat was wearing a new yellow collar to accessorise his black-and-white tuxedo coat.

'He lost the last one,' said the receptionist.

My guess is that this 'loss' was intentional on Arti's part.

~ ~ ~

Soon I would be catching another bus, this time for the Peloponnese, but there was time for an early morning walk. My destination? Filopappou Hill. On my first visit to Athens, I'd summitted this hill to find the structure I suspected was the 'temple' my mother and grandmother had 'tried to push over' — and hoped to Hades that Mum's cryptic diary entry wasn't to be taken literally — but I hadn't found the shrine to the Muses.

Julius Antiochus Philopappos was a Roman consul, Syrian by birth, who served the citizens of Athens in the second century. His memorial, cresting the hilltop that bore his name, was impressive. It was still standing inside its sturdy enclosure, forever protected from little old ladies who might be tempted to give it a shove.

The last time I was here, I wanted to take an unplanned detour along the ridgeline to a viewpoint over Piraeus and the Aegean Sea beyond. But I had an unsettled feeling about three men I spotted on the lonely hilltop. My suspicion was almost certainly unfair but, ever since a rape attempt in my twenties, I prefer to trust my instincts. Avoiding any potential threat, however unlikely, I headed straight to the Philopappos monument and then returned to the Acropolis.

In sticking to the most direct route, I missed finding a site more ancient than the tribute to Philopappos. Long before Athenians named this hill after the Roman consul, they called it the Hill of the Muses. Somewhere among its network of crisscrossing pathways was a shrine to the nine goddesses of the arts. Not seeing it had been a mild regret.

Now, as the soft silver of morning brightened to blue, I took the ridgeline track to the lookout at its furthest point, perched high above the city. I twice encountered lone male walkers, but this time I sensed no danger, and the ramble in the serene solitude of the hills filled me with peace. On my way down the hill, I tried a few false trails before locating the one leading to the Muses' shrine. It was just metres from the path I'd chosen last September. Musing about my newfound passion for writing — and hoping for inspiration from Calliope, Clio and Thalia, the goddesses of epic poetry, history and comedy — I picked a yellow daisy and placed it among the sacred stones. The art of writing has evolved since ancient times and none of these Muses was an exact fit for my story, but a little supernatural assistance couldn't hurt.

When I'd walked this hill before, I'd cradled a hollow pit in my belly where my passion for life should have been. But perhaps the Muses had been looking out for me, even if my sense of self-preservation had hindered me from paying respect to their shrine. After all, they were female, too. They would have understood why women sometimes compromise with caution.

Maybe that was when they took pity on me and gave me what I truly needed, rather than what I sought: a dream that I was writing my first book. I'd thought it was travel that was missing from my life, but recovering my wanderlust was only a step on my journey to fulfilment. It was writing that would transform my reality, that would challenge me in ways I couldn't have imagined. *The trouble with writing*, I often ponder, *is that when I started, I thought I was really good at it.* Instead of being the amusing pastime I'd anticipated, the discipline of the craft became a compass that guided me to sail past old horizons, to push through the claustrophobic borders that contained my middlescence.

~ ~ ~

Today's commute began with a bit of taxi confusion when I exited the hotel between a woman and her less punctual husband, both with strong South African accents. The driver, presuming we were travelling together, made to load my luggage into the boot. When I explained I'd be travelling to Nafplio by bus, he shared with me that he loved Nafplio and would be going there on his own holidays in July. He said to be sure to visit the Italian gelateria and, when I asked how to find it, he insisted, 'Everybody in Nafplio knows the Italian who makes the perfect gelato. All you need to do is ask.'

The metro took me as far as Omonia, but I still had to catch the local bus, number 051, to get to Kifissos Bus Terminal and its long-distance coaches. As I walked from the metro station to the bus stop, temptation drew up in the form of another taxi disgorging its passengers right in front of me. Remembering my awkward balancing act on the crowded twenty-minute bus ride to Kifissos the previous year, I threw frugality to the winds. This time, I'd take a cab as far as the coach terminal.

At first, the driver didn't understand where I wanted to go. 'My English,' he apologised with a timid smile, 'she is not beautiful.' I wished I had the Greek to tell him how wrong he was.

~ ~ ~

The coach ride was uneventful, apart from one delicious moment when classical and pop cultures met:

6 June 2017
The irony of Bonnie Tyler's *Holding Out for a Hero* belting out on the bus's sound system as we pass a sign to ancient Mycenae.

The Nafplio Grand Sarai was in the Old Town, just a short walk from the bus station. It was fancier than my usual fare, with elaborate timber staircases that were artworks in their own right. As in Corfu, the time constraints of organising this trip on short notice had prevented my customary thorough search for good-quality, cheap accommodation. My lodgings were still excellent value for money, though, compared to even the most characterless budget chains in Australia. I luxuriated in my airy corner room, leaning out of the windows to photograph a Greek Orthodox chapel on one side and a Catholic church overlooking the hotel terrace on the other.

There was no time to waste. Although I had two and a half days to spend here, I had resolved to fit in visits to Mycenae and Epidavros. Both were on bus routes out of Nafplio but, regrettably, in opposite directions. Grabbing my water bottle sling, I set out to explore what I could of the town.

My first stop was the chapel I'd seen from my window. Not only was it dedicated to Agios Spyridon, over whose sainted relics I had bowed so deferentially in Corfu, but it was once the setting of a historic drama. Here, on *this* nondescript church step leading onto *that* narrow lane, was the scene of the bloody 1831 slaying — by both pistol and dagger — of Count Ioannis Kapodistrias, the first governing head of state of modern Greece. A painting in the church portrayed the assassination in graphic detail.

Three minutes' walk took me to a majestic arch guarding the base of a rocky mound that glowers over Nafplio. The knowledge that I'd resolved to scale the outcrop's heights made it even more intimidating.

The stone steps to Palamidi climb the hot rockface in a relentless zigzag, but the spectacular views over the Old Town and the Argolic Gulf make for plenty of surreptitious rest stops disguised as photographic opportunities. I took multiple shots of the little island fortress of Bourtzi emerging from the blue in the middle distance and then diminishing in size as the stairs mounted higher and higher.

The first gateway proved deceptive. There was a lot further to climb: it was more than a thousand upward steps to the highest point of the fortifications sprawled across the summit. At last, red-faced and sweaty, I arrived at the entrance to the fortress and handed over eight euros.

A sign described Palamidi, a vast complex of eight bastions two hundred metres above the harbour town, as 'an achievement of military architecture', though perhaps not a complete martial success: 'It was built at the end of the second period of Venetian rule (1711–1715), but was conquered by the Turks before completion, and came into Greek possession on November 29, 1822, when the chieftain Staikos Staikopoulos and 350 elite troops invaded the fortress, forcing the Turkish garrison to surrender without a fight.'

This brief resumé gave the impression that the citadel fell rather short in its defences. It did, however, later become an effective prison for those on death row or sentenced to life imprisonment. Remembering the pretty church of Agios Sostis I visited on my first trip to Athens last year, and its unusual history, I wondered if this was where they beheaded King George's would-be assassins in 1898.

In Saint Andrew's Bastion, the oldest in the fortress, a green tree reached towards the blue sky. It was almost the sole splash of colour amid a network of sand-coloured stone steps, stone ramps, and stone arches in high stone walls. A few metres past this tree, a gloomy door gaped like a toothless mouth between two barred-window eyes. A cheerful row of red pots holding a bounty of basil offset the ominous effect.

The door led to the tiny chapel of Agios Andreas. Its vaulted ceiling was stained with damp, and the tiled floor started with a neat black-and-white chessboard pattern that devolved into chaos a dozen rows back from the wood-panelled altar. The walls were mottled plaster, sparsely decorated with icons. The most ornate feature was a gilded stand, holding two lit tapers in a shallow dish of sand.

I'm not a religious person. But my parents were, and I often light candles for them in places of worship around the world. This honours their memory, and my upbringing, in a way that would have meant something to them. Once, in the holy Hindu city of Haridwar, I sent a small flame

— nestling among colourful flowers and cupped in a green leaf — down the rushing waters of the Ganges. But, usually, it's the slender wax tapers found in Christian churches that I light, and they tend to be for my mum. My father gets an occasional candle, though, in places he would particularly like. This one was for him.

He was a staunch Roman Catholic, an honourable and sometimes stern character. We had little in common apart from our insatiable love of reading. Oh, and the shared stubbornness that made my adolescence a tough time for us both, especially when I left the church that was such a critical component of my parents' lives and moral systems. He was sixty-nine when we lost him to a fatal heart attack. I, the youngest of his six children, was twenty-three.

Dad had been a teenaged soldier with the Allies in the closing years of the Second World War. He traversed Egypt in an armoured car and — if his anecdotes over the years told the true tale — experienced Allied-occupied Italy through a series of bars. His humorous dinner-table stories of his escapades there seemed a sharp contrast to his strict behaviour when I knew him, and I was never sure how much of what he related was tongue-in-cheek. He was a man who managed to balance his often-austere demeanour with a wonderful sense of humour.

He marched into Naples the day after the fighting ended. There was no prompt return home, though. He was stationed there for more than a year, and he and his mates were assigned to aid Italian authorities in preventing the smuggling of olive oil through the Alps. When he finally got to return to South Africa, he landed in Cape Town, caught a train across the country to Johannesburg and, without telling a soul he was on his way, took a bus home to the suburb of Orange Grove. In shades of Odysseus, his dog was waiting for him at the bus stop.

Despite such adventurous travel in his youth, the sole overseas trip he took as a post-war adult was a visit to the United Kingdom with my mum in 1981 to get to know their young grandson.

I have childhood memories of us playing chess, with Dad bearing a hefty handicap. He'd decide how many of his pieces I could remove before the game began, and I'd choose which they'd be, from the ranks of pawns, bishops, even the queen. Only his king was immune from this pre-game cull.

These pieces were from his wartime set, and he kept them folded in the yellowing handkerchief he'd carried in North Africa and Europe. Although I was only little and never took to the game, I recognised that he was sharing something special. The air was rich in ritual whenever he slid open the splintered wooden box to take out this hanky-wrapped bundle of pawns and bishops, rooks and knights.

With his keen interest in military history, the fortress of Palamidi would have fascinated him. He'd have prayed for lost comrades in this little chapel, its bare walls soaked in the last desperate entreaties of bygone soldiers. Then, stiff with arthritis, he'd have stalked through the hilltop undergrowth, his knobbly knees visible beneath long khaki shorts, as he relived the battles of long ago.

~ ~ ~

You have to go out into the sunshine and up a flight of stairs to get to the spooky dungeon hidden deep in the wall beside the church. If you take the time to read the sign, you'll learn that it's been called the 'Prison of Kolokotronis' since the early twentieth century, but that it was actually more likely to have been a powder magazine. A roped-off queueing area bears testimony to its often-high numbers of visitors.

Alone in this part of the castle, I was free to creep into the small space, with no hurry to make way for anyone else. The door was so low that I had to bend double to enter. There was a short passageway — just a step or two — and then a shallow drop into a crude antechamber. A second doorway was again so low that, when I sat on the threshold, my head was barely ten centimetres below the lintel. Rough stairs descended further into a claustrophobic vault with scorched walls and a floor that was just earth packed between ribs of exposed rock.

The air was stale and dank, disturbed only by the *plink* of moisture dripping onto stone. The walls were icy cold.

For the sake of the captives of old, I hoped this was indeed a storeroom for gunpowder, and not the prison cell it had become in popular legend.

Exiting into the sun's glare, I continued past parapets pierced with arrow slits peeping out at magnificent views over the city of Nafplio. Along this path stood the Bastion of Miltiades, named after a hero of the ancient Battle of Marathon. This was the true prison of Theodoros Kolokotronis, a leader of the Greek War of Independence and a supporter of the same Count Kapodistrias who was ambushed at the little church next to my hotel.

Kolokotronis once rode to victory at Palamidi, a ride memorialised by a statue in Nafplio's town square, so it was ironic that, when he was condemned to death for treason in 1834, his captors imprisoned him here until his pardon a year later. In 1840, and for the next eighty years, Palamidi's Bastion of Miltiades became a prison for others awaiting execution or serving life sentences. I meandered in and out of its rooms, only to receive a karmic payback for my morbid voyeurism when I slipped on a doorstep and fell, scraping the skin off the meaty part of my palm in a bloody, stinging graze.

It took more than four hours for me to visit all eight bastions of Palamidi Fortress. I climbed to the furthest point I could reach, my perceptions heightened by the exertion of the hike. Historical connections glimmered all around, and the views across both land and sea shone with radiant glory as the late afternoon faded to evening. The fortress hadn't been crowded when I arrived and, by the time I got to the last two bastions, I had broken away from the main walking loop. I was alone.

Adventure, I believe, is wherever you happen to find it. You don't have to search for it in the rainforests of the Amazon or the sand dunes of the Sahara. It could be waiting for you wherever you take just a step outside your comfort zone. For me, this step was the first of seventeen disappearing into the gloom of an underground cistern. Aware I had left the tourist circuit behind, I knew that, if I fell, I might lie in the dark under the Bastion of Fokion until morning. At best.

I inched forward with care, but my fingers brushed silky spiderwebs when I reached out an arm to steady myself. I snatched my hand back, then kept it outstretched, not quite touching the cobwebbed wall but ready to grab for it if — worst-case scenario — I lost my balance. Two of my fears loomed at once: a not-unusual dread of heights and an extreme arachnophobia. Braving these primal terrors was quite different from the logical argument I carried out with myself each time I boarded a bus. It was the scariest thing I'd done in a while.

It was still light when I tackled the thousand stairs down the hill, and I was far too weary to stay up for dinner. I opened a bottle of Robola in my hotel room, and a vacuum-sealed pack of olives I'd bought on Kefalonia. The wine was lovely, but the briny olives were so nasty that I threw them away and did without any supper.

Breakfast was a different matter altogether. The usual spread was supplemented by delectable sweet and savoury pastries, including delicate spanakopita (spinach and cheese in filo) and unsweetened cakes of deep-fried dough reminiscent of South African vetkoek, stuffed with minced olives. I ate my fill, as the day was bound to be a tiring one. I was going to try, using the bus network, to visit both Mycenae and Epidavros.

CHAPTER TWELVE
A VISIT TO MYCENAE

MYCENAE IS REPUTED TO have been the home of King Agamemnon, the particularly unpleasant leader of the thirteenth-century BCE Greek campaign to lay siege to Troy, a kingdom in the land now known as Turkey. The catalyst for warfare had been the adulterous liaison between his sister-in-law, fair Helen of Sparta, and a Trojan prince named Paris.

In fact, Helen was Agamemnon's sister-in-law twice over. She was married to his brother Menelaus, and her sister Clytemnestra was Agamemnon's wife. Neither marriage was blessed with happiness and, according to Homer's epic poem *The Odyssey*, Agamemnon was still complaining about Clytemnestra from the shadowy underworld of the dead. As for Helen and Menelaus — well, we'll never know whether Helen left voluntarily or if Paris snatched her away against her will, but we do know that her seduction, or abduction, resulted in a brutal ten-year war to win her back.

Cynics might argue that the conflict was more about regaining Helen's fortune than her fabled beauty; Paris may have raided Agamemnon's treasury as well as his bedchamber. Unless the Greek invasion was about the geopolitical advantage held by Troy, which was perfectly located at the mouth of the Dardanelles to guard the juncture between Europe and Asia. When I eventually got to visit the likely site of the siege, years later, I was struck by how close it was to the First World War Turkish battlefields of Gallipoli, and how the strategic value of that strip of water has provoked so much bloodshed over the millennia.

The conflict may have had nothing to do with love, jealousy, or dowry. But whether it was because of her pretty features, or her wealth, or even if the warrior-politicians of the day just used her as an excuse, Helen's was 'the face that launch'd a thousand ships', as Elizabethan playwright Christopher Marlowe wrote in his tragedy, *Doctor Faustus*. These were Greek ships setting sail for Troy. Agamemnon waged a decade-long war against the Trojans that ended with Odysseus's cunning trick of hiding soldiers inside a hollow wooden horse. The siege ended when the gullible defenders of Troy took the horse for tribute, dragging it inside the city's fortified walls.

Now, the ruins of Mycenae's principal settlement encircle a scrubby knoll, working their way up to the acropolis at its crest. Sparse yellow grass grows over the mound that might well have been the centre of Agamemnon's kingdom, and the adjacent hills dwarf it on either side. Ominous thunder boomed as I neared the Lion Gate, and I overheard a guide tell her group, 'Zeus is talking to us.'

The gate guarding the acropolis bears what may be the oldest surviving relief sculpture in Europe: two thirteenth-century BCE lions, now headless, standing on their hind legs above a colossal stone lintel. Academics may argue over whether the events and characters of the Trojan War were factual or mythological but, if they *were* real, the heroes of legend would have tramped through this same gateway under which I now trod.

I walked around the impressive grave circle where nineteenth-century archaeologists discovered the golden death mask popularly known as the Mask of Agamemnon, which I'd seen in an Athens museum during my first Greek holiday. Then, I ascended to the acropolis and the building believed to have been Agamemnon's palace and, quite possibly, the site of his murder. In my favourite version of the tale, it was his vengeful wife Clytemnestra who snared him in his bath and then, as he struggled to escape her net, slaughtered him. Perhaps with the help of her lover, Aegisthus. Who, incidentally, was Agamemnon's cousin. Families, eh?

While Clytemnestra's methods are obviously to be deplored, it is hard not to empathise with her rage. Before going to war, Agamemnon had lured their daughter Iphigenia away with a false promise of betrothal to Achilles. Helen's face, it turned out, was not enough to launch the ships, which were trapped, becalmed, at harbour. Instead of marrying Iphigenia to a hero, her father sacrificed her to the goddess Artemis to secure the steady winds he needed to carry his boats to Troy.

Just as this thought slipped through my mind, a fresh breeze blew up, and a brief scattering of heavy raindrops fell from thunderous skies. I passed the ruins of houses, temples and the artisans' quarter before coming to steep steps leading into another cistern. This time, as I descended, there were a couple of fellow tourists thirty paces ahead of me, and I crossed paths with another on my return to the surface.

You can't tell where you're going, buried in the darkness, but the staircase led below the citadel walls to a dead end located outside the stronghold. This cramped space was the base of a shaft plunging eighteen metres underground. In structure, this cistern was nothing like the cavernous arched vault into which I had climbed at Palamidi. It was different, too, in that there was no sense of disuse, no danger of lying for hours or days among the spiders if I fell.

I wondered if these were the steps that controversial American author Henry Miller twice tried and failed to descend, once in the company of Lawrence Durrell. Describing the ordeal in his travelogue, *The Colossus of*

Maroussi, he imagined they led to a 'slimy well of horrors'. Of course, that was in 1939. The ambience may have been very different, then.

I left the acropolis with a satisfactory feeling of having completed the highlights, ticking all my boxes, but my most special memory of Mycenae still lay ahead.

Walking down the hill and over grass the pale colour of hay, away from the busier areas of the site, I came across a gaping hole in the ground. This was more than a random cavity. It was a circular tomb called a *tholos* that the Mycenaeans had dug into the hillside below. Thousands of years ago, the chamber of the tomb would have been topped by a curved roof shaped like an old-fashioned straw beehive, but now it lay open to the sky.

I scrambled down the slope to the base of the hill, where a long, straight path led to an imposing doorway. Inside, the walls stretched far higher than I could reach. Their intricate stonework was striking, and I crossed the *tholos* to examine the wall on the opposite side.

As I approached the centre, a powerful tramp of marching feet accompanied me. I froze, startled, and the following marchers halted too. I looked around, but there was no one there. I stamped a foot, and a single beat of myriad feet boomed across the *tholos*. I spoke, and my voice echoed. Despite having lost its roof in the thirty-five centuries since its construction, the *tholos* had an eerie resonance. The ground seemed to shiver with my steps, but surely that was an illusion caused by the wind and the weird sound effects... right?

The roof of the next beehive tomb was intact. This *tholos* was slightly bigger than the first, almost fifteen metres across its diameter, and its cupola soared high above my head. Sound had the same peculiar quality here, so I waited until there was nobody within earshot before chanting a drawn-out yoga 'Om' to enjoy the reverberation of the mantra, magnified under the dark dome.

CHAPTER THIRTEEN
NAFPLIO, WITH AN
AFTERNOON IN EPIDAVROS

THANKS TO SOME SNAPPY bus timetabling, I entered the Asclepieion at Epidavros a couple of hours later. This medical sanctuary was the legendary birthplace of Asclepius, the god of healing and the son of Apollo, for whom my Sri Lankan hospital was named. Epidavros was the greatest of hundreds of *asklepieia* throughout the ancient Greek and Roman world, like the one I'd visited at Butrint in Albania a few days before.

You can walk all over this vast haven of classical medicine: past the foundations of a hostel for the pilgrims of old and the remains of a banquet hall, temples, baths, wells and fountains. Water played a crucial role in the treatments offered here. Ritual bathing preceded a deep sleep in which Asclepius would come to the patients in dreams, sometimes accompanied by a sacred serpent, and visit health-giving miracles upon them. Diet, exercise, medication and even surgery supplemented these wondrous therapies, but credit for the cure went to the dream.

Epidavros is also home to a fine stadium with a tunnel from which athletes could make a glorious entry, just as football teams do today. The scent of pine trees infused the air of the arena, and cones and needles littered the rows of empty stone seats overlooking the abandoned track.

For all its history and sprawling size, the therapeutic sanctuary is not the drawcard for most modern travellers to Epidavros, many of whom never see its healing waters, temples and stadium. Instead, they come for the theatre. And I don't mean the inherent drama of the site. I'm talking about the actual open-air theatre. This outdoor auditorium could accommodate up to twelve thousand people in its heyday. Like the stadium, it was linked to the cult of Asclepius, with athletic, musical and dramatic competitions held in honour of the god.

After the pastoral peace of the ruin-strewn valley that lies before it, the theatre's impression of verticality gave a visual jolt. Its towering tiers were thinly populated by a smattering of weary souls in the late afternoon sunshine. People were taking turns at impromptu renditions of gospel, jazz, opera, a cappella sound effects, and even simple acts like tearing a sheet of paper to test the remarkable acoustics of the space. Some performances were superb, others not so much, but they all garnered applause. The faint whoops of appreciation from the fatigued audience seated far above may not have been the most exuberant, but they expressed a real sense of camaraderie.

As my fingers probed the lichen spreading across my stone seat in the very top row, my tired eyes rested on the distant blues, greens and golds of the landscape. An old man sang an Italian aria in a shaky tenor, followed by a choir of African American travellers singing *Worthy is the Lamb*. It struck me that, in this moment, the people around me were creating potent memories. They would take them back to every corner of the world and mull over them at random intervals for years to come. It was hard to drag myself away.

Worn out, hungry and increasingly anxious that I might have missed the last bus to Nafplio, I waited a long time alone at an unmarked stop. When it finally appeared, it was such a relief that I forgot to be frightened.

~ ~ ~

By cramming in excursions to both Mycenae and Epidavros the previous day, I had gifted myself an easy last day in Nafplio.

I began with the acropolis of Ancient Tiryns. This was a bit of a duty visit as I was starting to feel 'all ruined out', as can happen after weeks of traipsing around museums and archaeological remains. Tiryns is not as visually impressive as its sister-site, Mycenae, but together they make up a World Heritage Site. As it was only five kilometres from my hotel, I couldn't allow myself to miss the opportunity to see where Heracles — better known by his Roman name of Hercules — was sent by Delphi's oracle. This was the launchpad for his fabled Twelve Labours.

Tiryns boasts Cyclopean walls similar to those you can see in Mycenae. Their stone blocks are so massive that the Ancient Greeks believed it must have been the one-eyed giants of their legends, the Cyclopes, who put them in place. The second-century Greek geographer Pausanias wrote of Tiryns: 'The wall, which is the only part of the ruins still remaining, is a work of the Cyclopes made of unwrought stones, each stone being so big that a pair of mules could not move the smallest from its place to the slightest degree. Long ago, small stones were so inserted that each of them binds the large blocks firmly together.'

Imagine! Nineteen hundred years ago, these walls were already so ancient that the secret of their construction had been lost in the mists of mythology.

If you walk up to the high plateau of Tiryns, you can wander around the footprint of the citadel. There was no signage, and although my *Lonely Planet* had given me the heads-up to buy a booklet at the admission kiosk, its detailed descriptions of archaeological finds and architectural features did little to help me relate to the people who'd once lived here. Maybe it was the fault of my ruins fatigue, but the connection to the past I had felt in Mycenae and Epidavros eluded me.

~ ~ ~

Back in Nafplio, I passed a red-painted shrine outside the fire station and a man selling fresh garlic from a toddler's pushchair in a park, then ambled through the Old Town down to the waterfront. My goal was to catch a boat to the island fortress of Bourtzi, which sits just six hundred metres out to sea. This was the little castle that had steadily diminished in size as I'd climbed to the bastions of Palamidi two days before.

On the way, I came across a small shop festooned with Italian flags both inside and out, reminding me of the Athens taxi driver's insistence that 'everybody in Nafplio knows the Italian who makes the perfect gelato.' Sure enough, this was the Antica Gelateria di Roma, filled with colourful fruit, exotic bottles of liqueur and tray upon tray of creamy goodness. Ice cream isn't one of my usual vices, but I indulged in a small cup for the sake of the enthusiastic driver and the sheer flamboyance of the little shop. Not being a connoisseur, I can't give an educated verdict, but the cool, sweet treat lifted my energy after the morning's warm walk.

When I reached the waterfront, a sign told me the next boat to Bourtzi would leave *yesterday* at 11.00 a.m. I consoled myself with a massage at a pretty salon called Panta Rei, from a woman wearing the twin of my turquoise Greek goddess outfit, but in spotless white. The salon's brochure billed this as an 'Ancient Greek Massage'. I don't know the basis for this claim, but the masseuse had strong, skilled hands, and my backpack-carrying shoulders were grateful.

A shop flaunting images from Antoine de Saint-Exupéry's classic novella *Le Petit Prince* grabbed my attention. Called *Mikros Prigkipas*, which is Greek for 'Little Prince', the store was bursting with a tempting array of wares. Everything from clocks to musical instruments to kitsch ornaments — which were somehow charming amid the colourful cacophony of merchandise — spilled from its shelves. An intricate model of a fire engine caught my eye, and the shopkeeper climbed into the window display to retrieve it for me. He bubble-wrapped it, but I still took it straight to my room, where I swathed it in layer upon layer of garments and stowed it securely in my luggage, determined to get it home to Adam in one piece.

Bags packed, tummy full after a sadly unappetising late lunch of greasy lamb and stale chips, I glanced out of the window. It was late afternoon, but there was a little daylight left, and I hadn't yet visited the Church of the Transfiguration of the Saviour next door.

A few steps took me from the hotel to a marble panel mounted on the stone church wall, where I read that the building had been an eighteenth-century Ottoman mosque.

The engraved words told me it had been consecrated as a Catholic church in 1840, and that 'Philhellenes' of 1821 bones are kept in the crypt'.

The date of 1821 was significant. Greek Independence Day is celebrated on 25 March each year, commemorating the start of the 1821 revolution against the Ottoman Empire. The national struggle had waxed and waned over hundreds of years, but it was this eight-year War of Independence that finally led to the modern state of Greece. And it was during this war that philhellenism — foreign support for the national cause, based on a deep love for Greek culture — reached its peak. It attracted idealists from around the world, including many literary personalities.

The most famous philhellene was Lord Byron, the English poet, who died on the Greek mainland in 1824. Others came from as far away as America. The United States, having fought its own revolution within living memory, fostered great sympathy for the cause of Greek independence. I wondered about these particular philhellenes whose bodies lay under the church. *Where did* they *come from? When they arrived on the Peloponnese in 1821, ready to fight for the freedom of Greece, was that the first time they set foot on Greek soil? Were they hardened veterans of war who knew exactly what they were in for? Or enthusiastic youth with no concept of their own mortality, chasing a glorious adventure? And did their families ever find out how they died, or where their bones rested?*

The engraved words also explained the antique water tap and stone basin set into the wall at the foot of the stairway leading first up to my hotel and then further up to this church. There was a plaque there too, bearing old Turkish script. I understood, now, that the tap and basin would have been for ritual washing before prayers in the days when Muslims worshipped in this building, before it was converted into a church.

I spent a few minutes in the church and then, eyes down to avoid staring at the scrawny old man hunched over his book on a neighbouring balcony, looking for all the world like a shirtless Henry Miller, I spotted a hefty metal trapdoor set in the ground outside. It was standing open, and stone steps led to a simple crypt chapel. An automatic overhead light flicked on as I descended. There were no philhellenes' skeletons in sight, and it wasn't scary at all.

CHAPTER FOURTEEN
NAFPLIO TO POROS, WITH A
PILGRIMAGE TO HYDRA

A PRE-DAWN START TOOK ME on a three-bus journey from Nafplio to Galatas, the mainland town opposite the island of Poros.

The first bus dropped me and a large, taped-up cardboard box near the turn-off to Epidavros. It was 6.20 a.m. and deserted, but the driver told me in broken English to wait five minutes. Five minutes can feel a boring long time when you're standing at the side of a quiet road, so I examined the carton. Its label, 'Galatas' in Greek script, was reassuring. The box itself was more intriguing, printed with the outline of a flying-saucerish contraption below the English words 'PET DOME LIDS'. An initial theory, UFO components, I rejected as farfetched. My best deductive efforts led me to conclude that the box contained spare parts for some type of cat-carrier, but a later Google search informed me that the contents were the epitome of banality: the bulbous plastic lids for disposable drinking cups.

A minibus pulled up at 6.27 a.m., but its friendly driver explained that this was not my ride. 'Not to worry,' he said, 'your bus will come in five minutes, maybe less.' I was dubious, but the Athens-bound coach arrived three minutes later.

By a quarter to seven, the mysterious package and I had both boarded a third and final bus to take us to Galatas. This last exchange took place near a road sign announcing that we were fifteen kilometres from the Ancient Theatre of Epidavros. The sign's unexpected familiarity gave me a jolt: this was where I'd changed buses on my way to Limnisa the previous year, scrambling to get my baggage out of one and into the other. These bus swaps may have appeared random, but there was method in their seeming madness.

A pink sun was rising over a coastal panorama, but the driver was hawking up phlegm, spitting and coughing, spoiling the picturesque moment. I tried to keep my breaths shallow, in the hope I wouldn't catch whatever he had.

When the bus reached its destination, the PET dome lids and I parted ways. The carton would await its fate in Galatas, while I hurried to board the eight o'clock ferry to Poros along with that day's fresh produce and new-baked bread. Florian from Sto Roloi met the boat with his bright-orange quad bike, slung my laptop backpack over his handlebars, and loaded both me and my suitcase behind him. With my dodgy arm resting on the delicately balanced luggage and my good arm loosely clasped around Florian's belly, I pretended to be an old hand at quad bike riding, instead of this being an exciting new experience. He took me the short distance into town to leave my bags at the Sto Roloi office until my apartment, the Little Tower, was ready for check-in.

I had come to Poros for three reasons. First, a practical one: it was a convenient point from which to get to my final Greek destination, a direct ferry ride away. Second: this was one of the three islands my mother had visited in 1978. Third: from here it would be easy to make a day trip to another island where my mother's boat had docked. Her notes on Hydra were far more evocative than her brief description of Poros, where all she said was that she'd 'Paddled in puddles & took photos'. As soon as I was free from my luggage, I bought a ticket for my second ferry ride of the morning, this time to the island of Hydra.

~ ~ ~

Henry Miller visited Hydra in the 1930s, describing the town huddled around its main harbour as 'a pause in the musical score of creation' in *The Colossus of Maroussi*. In *Sextet*, published more than three decades later, he spoke of the island as having been 'built by a race of artists... a dream born out of a rock.'

Hydra has long been renowned among Greeks for its pivotal naval role during the War of Independence against the Ottomans. It came to global attention in the 1950s, when it was the setting of the first Hollywood movie shot in Greece. *Boy on a Dolphin* starred a young Sophia Loren, making her 1957 Hollywood debut as a sponge diver caught up in the ethical dilemmas around the sale of historical artefacts. Iconic Aussie artist Sidney Nolan spent a season painting on Hydra in the fifties. In 1960, Canadian musician and poet Leonard Cohen, best known for his enigmatic song *Hallelujah*, moved to the island, where he met hard-living Australian writer couple Charmian Clift and George Johnston. The island became a creative haven sought out by artists from many lands.

Hydra's authorities have preserved its atmosphere by placing strict limits on building projects, and the island has a reputation for being almost entirely free of motorised vehicles. Cars are banned, and only a few emergency service and miniature utility trucks are allowed. In the Old Town itself, even bicycles are prohibited.

I had five hours until my ferry would leave Hydra, so I started with a leisurely search for a morning meal. After picking my way between a row of donkeys tied up on land and a line of boats bobbing at their harbour moorings, I found a café serving an English breakfast. It had been weeks since I'd tucked into a plate of fried eggs and crispy bacon, so I settled happily at an outdoor table. While waiting for my order, I re-read the relevant passage from my mother's diary.

> *Date* Thursday 19th
> *Place* Athens Aegina Poros Hydra
> *Weather* Rainy then Cool
> … Onto Hydra. Wandered through streets with Mom Father & Johnny. Donkey tied to tree. All houses closed. Drank beer. Thousands of cats. Walked up to cannons. Climbed down steps to sea. Back to boat at 4 & off once more…

I consulted my *Lonely Planet* and decided to walk up to the monastery of Profitis Ilias before it got even hotter than it already was, and then explore the port to find my mother's cannons. Navigating through the steep streets, I encountered quite a few cats sprawled across doorsteps and shady cobblestones, but not the thousands my mother had reported.

When I reached the upper edge of the cluster of buildings arranged around the harbour like an ancient theatre, I had a moment of false hope that I'd made it to the monastery. Greek script on the church's icon showed me my error: it depicted a different saint. So I set out in earnest on the long, hard slog up the hill, accompanied by the buzz of cicadas and a hint of equine dung in the air. Dogs were barking in the distance, interrupted by a persistent clanging like a cowbell. Gazing down past the terraced fields and the stone walls that trailed the hillside, I pinpointed the source of the sound: a donkey with a bell around its neck, picking its solitary way through cobbled backstreets in the village I'd left far below.

I climbed up and up, and more up, on an ever-changing path that was broad and gravelled in some places, narrow and paved in others. At last, I came across a heap of rocks someone had stacked into the rough shape of an armchair. It was a knobbly imitation of the real thing, but it was in the shade. I took a grateful seat.

This was where I met the young couple who'd been gaining ground on me for some time. Unusually cranky, I'd already decided to dislike them — their effortless progress in their skimpy sports gear made me feel unfit and frumpy, and the cheerful music playing from their phone was irritating — but they stopped to chat and turned out to be lovely. Greek tourists from Athens, they greeted the news that I was from South Africa with enthusiasm as the girl had travelled to Johannesburg and Cape Town, and the boy was planning a trip to South Africa for the coming August. They were a lot stronger, fitter and younger than me, and they laughed merrily when I encouraged them to go on ahead. I, by contrast, was a panting mess as I struggled along the switchback turns. Tracks through the pine forest showed that people had been taking shortcuts between the zigzag curves, but I avoided these. I didn't want to contribute to erosion. Also, to be frank, the path was steep enough as it was.

On one of my frequent breaks, my Fitbit measured my heart rate at 163 beats per minute; it was a painful knocking against my ribs. The heat was making me ill, and, uncharacteristically, there were moments when I came close to giving up.

Eventually, I arrived at a whitewashed gateway and a chapel. My elation soon evaporated: I had somehow come in the back way and was in the monastery's working area of donkeys, sheds and debris. It had taken two hours to get this far, although it seemed much longer. And there was a bit more *up* to go before I'd reach the heart of the monastery.

At approximately 500 metres above sea level, perseverance paid off. A walled courtyard crowned the summit, and the little enclosed church made for a striking scene, with dark brickwork mortared in broad bands of white. I climbed its steps and admired its gilded icons through a lattice.

The monastery has been here since 1813. Founded by a group of monks from Mount Athos and built on the site of an eighteenth-century chapel, it commemorates Ilias, the biblical prophet my parents knew as Elijah. There was even a link with my old friend, the revolutionary Theodoros Kolokotronis, whose prison I saw in Nafplio. He was jailed in the cells of this monastery, too, albeit for only four months in 1825.

There wasn't a monk to be seen. Even the tiny shop was unstaffed, with a slotted moneybox to receive honour-system payments for the merchandise on its shelves — each icon, bead bracelet, bar of homemade soap, religious book or packet of wild rose tea labelled with its price. A drinking fountain providing free chilled water was a thoughtful gesture.

The descent was easier than the way up had been, though it was hard on the knees. The heat was like a hammer and, since my mother had recorded in her travel journal that she drank a beer on Hydra, I resolved to do the same. But the scorching sun had given me a headache by the time I reached the harbour, so I gulped down a fresh orange juice instead. While sipping a second juice, served hipster-fashion in a glass jar, I recovered enough to observe my surroundings and, particularly, the many donkeys around the port.

Mum had described the weather during her island odyssey as 'Rainy then Cool'. *She was lucky*, I thought. When I'd arrived in Hydra at 10.00 a.m. it was already oppressively hot, with a marked difference in comfort levels between sitting in the shade or exposed to the glaring sunshine. It was now afternoon, and the same donkeys were still standing in the same despondent line, awaiting the tourist trade. It broke my heart to see them tethered in their long row in the sun.

No shade. No water.

I am not against responsible horse riding, and I'm sure there are lots of donkeys on Hydra with caring owners. And many of this island's famous 'donkeys' are in fact mules, resilient creatures of surprising strength, capable of carrying heavy loads without strain. Countless animals in the tourist trade all over the world suffer harsh conditions, though, and accountability belongs as much to those of us who pay for these interactions, without considering a mount's welfare, as it does to the operators who hire them out to make a living. It's sometimes hard to look beyond the obvious, when we're out having fun. *But,* I thought, *how difficult is it to notice whether an animal has shade and water on such a hot day?*

With the lack of motorised vehicles on Hydra, working animals are a fact of life. But, as I photographed a beast burdened with a bulky load of building materials, and another parked in the sun on an uncomfortable gradient, shifting its weight from one hoof to another, I felt sad for the donkeys of Hydra.

Things have got better, though. Years after my visit to the island, I came across an online photograph of the exact harbourside location where I had witnessed those unhappy-looking donkeys standing in the sun. The animals were still there, but this time they were shaded by a row of enormous white umbrellas. I couldn't see a trough of water in the photo, but I like to think it was there.

~ ~ ~

Rehydrated, I returned to my mission to trace my mother's footsteps. I'd seen Mum's cats — or, at least, some of them — and closed houses aplenty. In the monastery's yard, I'd met a donkey tied in the shadow of a tree. But I had yet to visit the cannons or climb steps to the sea.

I feared the cannons would be elusive, but the opposite was true. Hydra's harbour has an overabundance of them. I found three locations with multiple cannons and laid my hands on the black paint coating each of the old metal gun barrels, wondering which of them my mother might have touched four decades ago.

Below the main cannon site, a daunting set of steps led downward. At their head, an intimidating sign warned 'SWIMMING IS FORBITEN' in misspelled capital letters. These were the most likely contenders for the steps mentioned in Mum's diary, but the vertiginous staircase didn't make it all the way down to the water. Perhaps it was low tide? I wouldn't be able to reach the water from the narrow rocky shelf at its base, so I decided to choose a different stairway to descend in memory of my mother.

The next set of steps was worse. Disconnected slabs of uneven stone were suspended perpendicular to the seawall. Some of the treads were missing, like gaps in a yellowing set of dentures. The others hovered alarmingly above the boulders below. Shuddering, I made an executive decision that these were not Mum's steps.

The solid masonry of the third and fourth staircases was much less frightening. I clambered down both to make up for my earlier cowardice, only just managing not to drop my phone as I photographed my fingers dangling in the water.

~ ~ ~

Sto Roloi is the vision of a woman who describes herself, on her website, as an 'architect-hotelier'. Over the course of more than two decades, Marie Luise has acquired three properties on the island of Poros and restored them into charming accommodation for travellers. Of the Little Tower, a small apartment at the rear of a house named Anemone, she writes:

> ... on the properties' southeast corner was nothing but a ruin. It once had hosted the farmers' most valuable property: the donkey. In its place we constructed the 'Little Tower,' a cozy two room hide-away in the shape of a tower.

When I emailed Marie Luise to ask if she and Florian would mind being identified by name in this book, she replied, 'Our hidden lady, Jeanette, responsible for housekeeping, as well as Toni, our gardener, would certainly appreciate being mentioned as well. I hope you do not mind my referring to them, but we are a team of four who work together with love, fun and dedication.'

This close-knit team had transformed the rustic Little Tower into my personal sanctuary for the night. Its upstairs balcony looked out over the red terracotta roofs of the island to a scattering of sailing boats in the blue beyond. An internal spiral staircase led down from the bedroom and kitchenette to a cheerful sitting room and an exciting shower, with multiple jets of spraying water that revived my spirits after the morning's sweaty climb.

Despite my headscarf and sunscreen, and in spite of the invigorating shower, Hydra had left me with something approaching heat exhaustion. Although there were several hours of sunlight left, I stayed in my cool apartment, relaxing amid its soothing tones of blue, green and grey. I had an easy supper of *tiropita* (feta pastry) purchased from a bakery before I left Hydra and — after what felt like a gallon of chilled water — the remains of the Robola, which I had tipped into one of my screw-top water bottles and brought with me from Nafplio. And, after five days of slow reading, I finished *The Iliad*. Thank goodness; there's only so much sulking over wounded pride a woman can take! Who would have thought that one of the world's most enduring stories would be grounded in such spiteful petulance, or buried in tedious descriptions of the ornate armour protecting the victors or being stripped from the dead. That's seventy-four cents and quite a few hours I'll never get back.

My step tally for the day, according to my Fitbit, included an uphill climb equal to 139 flights of stairs. Almost all of those were on the way up to the monastery in baking heat.

I got there in the end, though.

CHAPTER FIFTEEN
POROS TO METHANA

MY FINAL DAY OF tourism kicked off with an expedition along a series of stairs and narrow lanes from the Little Tower down to the waterfront. Here, the local fire truck was being put to good use, its pink firehoses watering the trees on the wharf. I checked the timetable to reassure myself that the 3.30 p.m. ferry was running on schedule, and returned to my room to pack. This would be my last move between towns in Greece, and my next destination would give me an opportunity to focus on something rather different from the sightseeing I'd done thus far.

As I zipped my suitcase closed, I reflected that there was more than one layer of meaning in the word 'odyssey'. Homer's *The Odyssey* — which turned out to be a far more satisfying read than *The Iliad* — chronicled a ten-year voyage filled with adventures. But it was also a journey that ended in a homecoming. And in some ways, returning to Limnisa, the place that fostered in me the will to write, felt like coming home.

Florian's orange quad bike pulled up at check-out time, and he asked what I wanted to do with the rest of the day. I told him I was planning a carnivorous lunch before my upcoming week of vegetarianism. He asked if I was ready to eat now ('Why not?') and if I minded a longish walk into town afterwards ('Not at all!'). Grinning at my enthusiasm, he offered to drop me at Aspros Gatos, telling me that one of his relatives ran this waterfront taverna.

Travel folklore advises caution about recommendations for businesses run by family members, but Florian was solid gold. Aspros Gatos (Greek for 'White Cat') had been operating since 1909, and my *Lonely Planet* rated it as the best seafood taverna on Poros. I can't abide seafood, so I sidled past the octopus draped from an awning, sat at a table in a corner of the seaside terrace and ordered my last Greek moussaka. Sprinkled with pale cheese in a single-portion ceramic baking dish that was too hot to touch, it was exactly what I wanted.

Strolling along the curve of the Bay of Poros after the meal, I passed a crouching cat poised to pounce on an oblivious pigeon. A confusing hangover of guilt descended the moment I'd waved the bird away. Cats need lunch too.

While wandering Poros, I didn't find any puddles for paddling, as my mother had, but I did take plenty of photos. I climbed up to the *roloi*, the town's clock tower, and peered at the timepiece's intricate mechanism through a glass-shielded doorway. But, strangely weary, I chose to spend my last hour on the island sitting in a café near the wharf, drinking orange juice and reading, until Florian arrived with my suitcase to see me aboard the ferry.

~ ~ ~

The boat docked in Methana sooner than I'd expected, and I scurried to its gaping door through a haze of disorientation, grabbing my bags just in time to disembark. Even as I walked down the ramp, I was double checking that this was, in fact, my destination. The smiling face of Mariel, here to bring me home to Limnisa, dispelled my doubts.

I had first visited this writing retreat the previous September, having come across it quite by chance. Limnisa had generously welcomed me, a non-writer, into its community, and the company of authors and vibrant dinner conversations about their craft had fascinated me. As I left the retreat after that blissful week, I had no inkling I would ever return. Something must have seeded within me and germinated, though, because, a month later, I woke from a dream in which I was writing a book about my Greek holidays. I didn't know it then, but that was the moment that gave me purpose and steered my life onto a new course. It was the direction I needed to guide me out of my midlife malaise.

The instant I had that hunch that my Canadian trip might turn into another Greek one, I contacted Mariel to ask if I could come back to Limnisa. Returning to the place where it all started would mark a milestone in my writing journey. She replied that she had only one spot left: one room available for one week in my travel window. I laughed when she told me this would be during Limnisa's first-ever yoga retreat. When I'd been looking for yoga, I had found a writing paradise. Now that I sought a haven to write, my stay would include twice-daily classes run by Jolie, a Singaporean yogi whom Mariel had met while travelling in Sri Lanka.

The Sri Lankan connection seemed a good omen.

When we reached Limnisa, which was every bit as beautiful as I'd remembered, I greeted Philip and introduced myself to Jolie before settling into my room. I was increasingly out of sorts, though, and, by sunset, I guessed I was coming down with something nasty. Excusing myself from dinner, I slid between my bed's soft sheets. By morning, I was very ill indeed.

I'm not sure whether I caught the bug from the coughing bus driver two days before, but my malady was even more disgusting than his had been. Wracked with intermittent fevers, I nursed my aching muscles, dripping nose and razorblade throat as I toiled over my keyboard. The worst of it was that the ailment had settled in my lungs, a weak point since my asthmatic childhood. Aware that my ground-floor bedroom was adjacent to the outdoor yoga *shala* created for this retreat, I kept my shutters closed until after each morning's practice. It wouldn't be fair for my hoarse cough and occasional self-pitying groans to disturb the serenity of the yogis' surroundings.

With no Asclepius to bring a miraculous cure, I shut myself in my room for four days and nights: a self-imposed quarantine that — with '2020 hindsight' — now seems mind-bogglingly inadequate.

At first, I resented that this week, to which I'd so looked forward, had been marred by illness. Then, I acknowledged how lucky I was. My appetite was almost as robust as ever, so Mariel brought me lovingly prepared plates of food for lunch and dinner. For breakfast, I'd wait for the yoga class to start, then tiptoe out to help myself to bread, cheese, yoghurt and fruit. As soon as I heard the group leave the *shala* after their practice, I'd throw open my window to let in the fresh sea air. Sitting propped up in bed with my laptop on my knees, I could glance up any time I wished to see the beauty of the Saronic Gulf rippling before me. Inspiration was not hard to come by with such a view.

This is where I overcame the writer's block that had stalled me two chapters from finishing the first complete draft of *Unpacking for Greece*, and it is where some surprising themes worked their way into my manuscript. This is where the voices of the women in my family began to speak through my keyboard. My mother, my sisters, even my great-great-grandmother, they all clamoured to be heard.

The thoughts about my mum that had surfaced the last time I'd gazed at this view flooded through me, but this time the tide was rushing in over different sands. Back then, I'd been wanting to paint Mum with a brush of perfection. Now, I acknowledged that wouldn't be honest. *But who isn't flawed?* I reminded myself. *No one typing in this room, that's for sure.* It wasn't our shortcomings that mattered anymore. The words I wished she hadn't said, and those I wished I had, it was time to let them go. We'd been as unable to cross the ravine between us as I was when faced with the juddering walkway over the Corinth Canal, the first time I crossed onto the Peloponnese Peninsula. That might have changed, with time; we'd started to take careful steps towards each other in her final years.

A sad acceptance washed over me: at that time, and in that place, we'd both done the best we could.

It was also a relief to understand the reason for my exhaustion and uncharacteristic grumpiness on the trail up to the monastery on Hydra. It wasn't because I was a middle-aged frump. No, it was because my body was already incubating this wretched virus, and bunkering down for a battle.

When I recovered enough to emerge from my cocoon, I walked into the silky waters off Limnisa's pebble beach with a grateful sigh. I joined in the evening yoga sessions, but I'd come to appreciate both how illness had battered my body and how productive that crack-of-dawn writing time was, so I excused myself from the more strenuous morning practices.

Limnisa felt a bit forlorn without my companions from the last visit. I hadn't realised how strongly I'd identified the retreat with the time spent floating in the gulf with Pien, Anne and Petri, discussing their writing and speculating about what type of cake would appear for each day's afternoon treat. Their absence left me bereft, at first, though this may have been more a symptom of my illness and isolation than anything rational. Once I could share meals with the others, I warmed to this new, interesting mix of people. Everyone participated in both the yoga and their own creative endeavour, be it writing or drawing or something else. At the end of the week, though, when I calculated how much I owed my hosts by counting the checkmarks on the communal tally sheet for each glass of wine I'd poured, I noticed a pattern. Scanning the page, it was easy to guess who'd come here mostly for the yoga and who'd come mainly to write:

The yogis glowed with health, sharing their energy in the *shala*, eating in moderation and drinking little or not at all.

The writers' energy shone at the dinner table; we indulged in a couple of glasses to lubricate our chats about writing and the world, and went back to the buffet for seconds. After the others drifted away, I'd linger at the table with Toni, who was working in challenging circumstances in post-war Bosnia.

Our long conversations were sometimes amusing, sometimes harrowing, but always thought-provoking.

~ ~ ~

On my final full day in Greece, Mariel took me on a drive around the Methana peninsula. She runs this as a weekly Wednesday excursion during Limnisa's retreats but, last year, I'd arrived on a Wednesday evening and left the following Wednesday before sunrise, so I'd missed both opportunities. This week, there'd been a full carload booked to go and, besides, I hadn't been well enough for a hike in the heat. Knowing I'd missed out three times, Mariel offered to take me out alone on the Friday morning.

We stopped first at Makrilongos, a village built on the lip of a gently sloping crater cultivated as agricultural land. A friendly dog sniffed our feet as we watched Toni's departing ferry far below us, making its way to Athens via Aegina.

Mariel encouraged me to walk up through the character-filled village while she drove to the other side. Happy to agree, I wound my way between buildings pretty in their dilapidation, stacks of firewood propped against stone walls, and purple thistles crawling with bees. When I reached the top of this cluster of homes, her car was waiting. We drove around the quasi-island, stopping at the ruin of a deserted hamlet and at the whitewashed chapel of Agia Sotira. Outside the tiny church, two saplings wore humorous placards asking passersby for water and promising future shade in return. Mariel found a bucket and soaked the soil where the young trees stood.

Then we headed to our chief objective: Methana Volcano.

There are around thirty volcanoes on Methana, with the last confirmed eruption having occurred more than three hundred years ago. As we neared the lava dome that shares its name with the peninsula, I spotted road signs bearing in Greek script the word for 'volcano': *ifaisteio*. Surely this word derives from the name of Hephaestus, the god of volcanoes, fire, metals and blacksmiths? This was the last linguistic discovery of my trip, and it filled me with gladness.

We were lucky with the weather as we started our walk. It was noticeably cooler than it had been when we left the house. Wednesday's group had struggled with overheating to the point of nausea, so I counted myself doubly fortunate.

Greece had one more benediction to bestow on me. We were walking single file, with Mariel some distance behind, when she called to me to stop. She stretched out her arm, pointing to strange shapes that had appeared in the sea. We shaded our eyes and concentrated, at last making out a frolicking line of dolphins. They were so far away that their sinuous movements were more recognisable than the shapes of their barely discernible bodies.

It was a perfect moment.

Three-quarters of the way to the volcanic shaft, Mariel stopped to let me go on alone. I hiked through jagged grey and rusty red rock formations, with a tricky clamber up a tumble of boulders. At the summit — marked by the word 'VOLCANO' and a downward arrow in white paint on the rock — you can peer into a triangular chasm that I guessed was the volcano's vent plunging into the depths of the earth. And then there was a final breathless scramble so I could look over the edge. Cautiously holding my balance on the unsteady stones, I saw horizontal strata of cracked rock splintered into blocks, as if Hephaestus had built the gods' equivalent of a brick garden wall.

~ ~ ~

After an afternoon of repacking my bags and leafing through the contents of Limnisa's bookshelves, our last supper was a modest one. Unlike my first visit here, with writers arriving and departing daily and an always-full house, this sojourn had taken place in the closing week of Limnisa's spring season. Even before I'd emerged from my sickroom, individuals had been leaving day by day. Only Jolie, Bowie and I remained to share our farewell dinner with Mariel and Philip.

AFTER: REFLECTIONS

EPILOGUE
LOOKING BACK

I HADN'T PLANNED THIS SECOND visit to Greece, but the addition of ten destinations — first to discover in person and then to describe in writing — was only one of the surprises that appeared as I wrote my way through the chapters of *Unpacking for Greece* and then this far gentler sequel.

The 2016 trip was born from an irrational, desperate discontent. That journey gave me what I needed: a rough-edged sense of adventure as I confronted my anxiety. I found my *kefi*, my passion for life.

By my 2017 expedition, I was partway through drafting the first book in this series and aware that I would be marshalling new memories into written words. But that wasn't all that had changed. I also had the serenity to savour the details: the colour of the butterflies, the fragrance of the honeysuckle, the struggles of a fellow passenger to fight against sleep. I'm now content with who I am, and so this second trip was one of warm pleasure rather than overheated exhilaration.

The transformation in the texture of my writing, from one journey to the next, intrigued and delighted me. It mirrored my evolution from middle-aged fear to midlife fulfilment, and from reader to traveller to writer. Places I visited unearthed memories, which stirred the musings that found their way into these pages. Unanticipated events revealed areas of memoir I could explore.

The reasons for my unexpected 2017 trip, for example, allowed me to reflect on apartheid's violent death throes. I steered clear of the political minefields of the present day, though. Not only was I no longer sufficiently informed to comment on distressing current events, I also wasn't strong enough. There were at least two major acts of terrorism during this trip — one in Kabul, the other in London — and I am sure there were others that never made it into world news. I acknowledge it is a sign of my privilege that I could continue chronicling my travels without mentioning these attacks, but they were very much in my mind. In an era when so many exploit religion as a difference to be feared, I was soothed by the links and similarities between faiths I uncovered as I moved through Greece.

Again and again, I was drawn to the rituals of water. The gurgle of the mountain spring where pilgrims of old purified themselves before consulting Delphi's oracle echoed through the ages. So did the bygone bubbles in the basins near Ottoman-era mosques, the splash of the annual immersion of the Holy Cross in the Bay of Argostoli, the babble of the healing waters in Epidavros. I remembered the cleansing *mikveh* I'd seen the previous year in the Jewish museum on Rhodes, and how the decorated wooden bathing sandals in a nearby display case had looked so similar to the pair I'd seen outside a Muslim prayer room the day before.

I've always felt compelled to dip my fingers into new rivers, lakes or seas I've encountered on my travels, and this compulsion was potent on Hydra, where I imagined my mum might have done the same thing. I wonder if this urge is a relic from my childhood, when the holy water standing at the entrance to our Catholic church was a place to pause and make the sign of the cross, or whether it is something more primal, harking back to the waters of the womb.

My mother was always going to feature in this story, through the medium of her little red journal, but the chance sighting of a theatre poster in Corfu brought my father, momentarily, centre stage. Then he lurked in the wings to reemerge for an encore in Nafplio. Just as with my mother, my relationship with my father was uneasy while he was alive, and I moved out of the family home before my eighteenth birthday. Dad died when I was twenty-three, with my mother following four years later. Our worldviews had diverged dramatically as I grew from a wayward teenager into a headstrong adult, but the introspection of writing has helped me accept that, although we couldn't identify with each other's beliefs, my parents' efforts to support me were unflagging. It couldn't have been easy for them.

My sisters Jenny and Tassin, whose voices had spoken so strongly in *Unpacking for Greece*, returned in this second manuscript and Jenny brought along my brothers for a cameo appearance. And, as if it wasn't enough for my parents and siblings to stake their claim, a long-departed female ancestor demanded to have her say, too.

A question at a Kefalonian bus stop led to my great-great-grandmother's fleeting appearance. She was a formidable woman who left her descendants a precious gift: a handwritten record of her eight decades on four continents. The first time I ever saw my writing between real book covers, it was in an anthology called *Itchy Feet: Tales of Travel and Adventure*. My chapter braided my words with Grandma Gropp's to tell the story of her remarkable life. She was one of the brave pioneers who brought my family to South Africa amid the multifaceted brutality of colonialism. It took an insightful editor to point out that my niece Carly was part of Grandma Gropp's story. Carly was the other nomad in our family. She died in Hanoi in April 2019, just months after we danced together at the joyous occasion of Christopher and Karen's wedding. Since then, every word I've written has been for her.

In a book that begins in Cape Town, it's impossible not to reflect, for a page or two, on the unearned privileges that came with growing up white in apartheid South Africa.

The thing is, privilege is about more than material possessions. You can't measure it in absolutes. If my Aussie friends were to examine my childhood out of context, they wouldn't think we were particularly privileged. I was never in danger of going hungry, it's true, but it wasn't a luxurious upbringing. We had a big house, but that was because we were a large, extended family: a single-income family, and it was a moderate income at that. We all shared bedrooms, and we'd be ousted from those rooms for days or weeks to accommodate unexplained guests. These were usually women and children who, I realise with adult hindsight, were seeking refuge from domestic abuse and found a temporary sanctuary with my parents through their church.

The little luxuries I take for granted today were few. Fizzy drinks were something that happened at Christmas. Single-serve tubs of yoghurt and other such frivolities never entered our home. My siblings still laugh about how my brother practiced the daily deception of squashing the soft centre of his thick-cut sandwich slices flat and then filling the indentations with peanut butter. But the joke is a sad one because my mother's bewilderment — at how quickly the peanut butter jars would empty — and dismay — at how replacing them would blow out her careful groceries budget — were real.

I am sometimes overwhelmed by how privileged my new life in Australia has become, with the social security I never had before, the standard of free health care, the generous leave provisions, enough income to travel, and the countless other advantages that have come to me in this lucky country. In fact, though, my existence has been laced with privilege since before my birth. As a white South African, everything I had — from the light in my bedroom that came on with the flick of an electric switch, to the comfortable teacher-to-student ratio in our school — came to me as a direct result of it being denied to someone else. I might not have asked for apartheid, but I benefitted from it every single day. And, with the ongoing effects of the opportunities that were open to me in my youth, I still do.

That's the thing about privilege that comes from systemic injustice. It's not about how much we have, it's that others don't.

~ ~ ~

Serendipity is a lovely word, isn't it? It's one of those delicious sounds, like Santorini. The *Collins English Dictionary* tells me that 'serendipity is the luck some people have in finding or creating interesting or valuable things by chance.' It is a happy synchronicity, and I stumbled across it all over Greece.

I'll never forget the morning when a tour guide in Athens, standing on a path my mother walked in 1978, tore a page from a notebook decorated with an image of Petra, the place

Mum yearned to visit above all others. Or when, on Corfu and partway through Gentill's Hero Trilogy, I happened on the information that Corfu was once the land of the Phaeacians she described. Or when I spotted a *Don Camillo* poster just weeks after I'd purchased the only *Don Camillo* book I own, decades after reading the series from my father's shelves. Or that I found a community of writers when planning a yoga holiday, and a yoga retreat when signing up for a writing hideaway. At the very same place.

Even while labouring over this book, there have been marvellous moments of serendipity. Some were simple discoveries, like learning that my father, my mother, and I had each visited Naples, separately and at decades-long intervals. Others were quite astonishing.

Like when I borrowed the *Lonely Planet Sri Lanka* from the local library here in Australia to check a specific memory: that it was in this guidebook I'd come across the recommendation, more than ten years before my Greek odysseys, to set out at 2.00 a.m. to climb Sri Pada. My own travel-worn copy was packed in a box in Megan's spare room in Cape Town, but the library held an edition from the same year in its collection.

Our librarians keep reserved books on a separate shelf, with the borrowers' names on reservation slips poking haphazardly out from between the pages. I'm a frequent user of this service, and I usually remove the slip of paper as soon as I get home, tossing it straight into the recycling bin. This time, I didn't. Which was lucky, because when I got around to opening the book a week later, I discovered the reservation slip, like a carefully inserted bookmark, at precisely the page I needed to check.

Or when I was searching in vain for the spelling of a half-heard Greek word from my second trip and the significance of a religious feast day I encountered during my first. When scouring the Internet failed to turn up the answers, I put out a random request for help in a large Discworld-themed Facebook group with thousands of Terry Pratchett fans from all over the world:

> 16 July 2017
> Any Greek members who wouldn't mind me asking some trivial questions (fact-checking for a book I'm trying to write)?
> 1. Is there a synonym of θάρρος that sounds something like the English word 'courage'?
> 2. What is the significance of the date 14 September in the Greek Orthodox calendar?

I received a quick and helpful response from an Athenian named Dimitra. In thanking her, I sent a message with the single paragraph from Chapter Three that included the word she'd taught me. Dimitra replied, 'Are you talking about Ayios Demetrios Loumbardiaris (tiny, tiny church on Fillopapou hill)? If so, I live almost right next door. So serendipity.'

In case you're wondering, I didn't remember she used the word 'serendipity' until I scrolled back through our messages, a few moments before transcribing her response onto this page.

And how serendipitous it is to discover that the word itself comes from *Serendib*, a long-ago Arabic name for the island once called Ceylon. Today, this island is known as Sri Lanka.

BUT WHAT ABOUT AEGINA?

You may have noticed that there was one place my mum visited that wasn't included in the itineraries of either my first book, *Unpacking for Greece*, or my second, *Repacking for Greece*.

It took another six years before I was able to visit the island of Aegina.

Read on to find out more.

But first…

Sign up to *Journeys in Pages*, my free email newsletter for readers, travellers and writers. Subscribers receive exclusive access to additional bonuses, including a fun online jigsaw puzzle and the story of my trip to Peru with my sisters and niece.

www.sallyjanesmith.com/newsletter

Enjoyed this book?
Please leave a review or star rating wherever you found it — even one short sentence makes more of a difference than you might think.

Want to see or hear more?
Visit **www.linktr.ee/SallyJaneSmith** for heaps of Greek-themed treats, including gorgeous photos, podcasts and puzzles.

Interested in helping an author out?
Ask your local library to stock the *Packing for Greece* series.

Belong to a book club?
Take a look at **www.sallyjanesmith.com/book-clubs** for more information.

Searching for a community of like-minded readers and writers who love memoirs in general and travel narratives in particular?
Join the friendliest group on Facebook, *We Love Memoirs.*

BONUS CHAPTER
AEGINA, MAY 2023

TWENTY-NINE DAYS INTO A six-week journey through Greece, I towed my suitcase off the ferry, the bag's wheels rattling over the ridges of the metal ramp. A last little bump brought me down onto the smooth paving of the wharf, metres from the tiny church of Agios Nikolaos Thalassinos that has graced Aegina's harbour for four centuries. I'd seen the whitewashed chapel before, but never from the ground — both previous sightings were from the deck of a ferry carrying me from the Peloponnese Peninsula to Athens.

My mother would have come across this chapel, dedicated to the patron saint of sailors, when she and my gran visited Greece with a group from their church in October 1978. They would almost certainly have ducked inside its dark doorway trimmed in blue paint. Mum was on an excursion that packed three island visits into one rainy day, so she wouldn't have had time to venture far from the port. Her diary entry for Thursday 19 October doesn't record much more for this stop than that she 'went walking on Aegina' and, bewilderingly, 'Chased Hen.'

I hope she didn't catch it.

If I had to take a guess, I'd say her walk would have taken her to the Temple of Apollo with its broken column that stabs up at the sky, visible from the port and less than fifteen minutes away. I'd found budget accommodation that promised a view of this solitary stone pillar, so I set off on the road she might have trodden, pulling my suitcase behind me.

I'd traced my mother's footsteps in Athens, Poros and Hydra on previous trips to Greece, but this was the first time I'd been able to fit in a stay on Aegina. I would have a day and a half on the island. *Should be enough*, I thought, uncharacteristically downplaying a destination's potential. *After all*, I assumed, perhaps incorrectly, *most foreigners, if they even come to Aegina, probably take the same three-island day trip as my mum and her friends.*

It's a bit embarrassing, now, to admit I hadn't put much thought into this brief island stopover. All my planning had been wrapped up in the three main segments of the grand Greek adventure I'd booked to celebrate the release of *Unpacking for Greece*: two weeks of solo travel through the majesty of Crete, another fortnight exploring the romantic Cyclades with Adam, and a final sojourn at a writers' retreat on the Peloponnese.

Aegina was to be a pause between beats, a chance to catch my breath between leaving Adam in Athens and joining the creative community of writers at Limnisa. I'd visit Apollo's temple and, after reading Grant Ginder's novel *Honestly, We Meant Well*, I was keen to see the Temple of Aphaia. But I knew little about either of these landmarks, and nothing at all about the rest of the island.

~ ~ ~

When I checked in to Kalokenti Studios, the owner, Stavroula, glanced at my scuffed hiking boots. 'Do you like walking?' she asked. And just like that, I was on my way to Paleochora and a strong contender for my most precious memory of Greece.

Well, I say, 'just like that,' but in fact it involved me nodding through a cascade of half-understood instructions and then rising in the dark, next morning, to catch the dawn bus to an unmarked stop outside Moni Agios Nektarios.

I'd visit this monastery later. For now, I'd follow my landlady's directions. 'Go behind the monastery,' she'd said. 'Then walk up the hill. There are signs.'

The truth is, I didn't really know why I was climbing this steep incline. Stavroula's tale was filled with pirates, and villagers fleeing their homes to escape the slave trade, and 365 churches, one for every day of the year. Barbarossa was in there, somewhere. But I'd been travel-weary and had only caught the merest gist of her story. As I gazed upward, though, something shifted in my mind, and the rocky hillside resolved into a pattern of tiny chapels tracing the slopes. They were stone against stone, not easy to see from afar, but the more I looked — and the closer I climbed — the more I found them... *everywhere*.

The word 'pirate' may sound glamorous to those of us who grew up with *Treasure Island* and *Peter Pan*, but the reality was far more brutal than even the Grimmest fairy tale. Brutal enough that the people of Aegina fled inland, far from their trade routes and fishing grounds. They built this settlement as a haven from ninth-century marauders, and they stayed for a thousand years. When the seas — and those who rode them — became less threatening, the islanders returned to the coast. And the buildings of Paleochora fell away to nothing.

Except for the churches.

There aren't 365 churches on this hill today, and possibly there were never quite that many. But almost three dozen still stand in testament to this high-ground refuge of long ago. And in testament to the faithful who come, each saint's day, to kiss an icon, to light a candle, to say a prayer.

For hours I wandered, scrambled and climbed from one tumbledown house of worship to another. A couple were not much more than four broken walls, open to the skies and overgrown with a profusion of cheerful daisies and blood-red poppies. Most were simple chapels, their chessboard floors swept clean, a mop and bucket in a corner by the door, and a few beloved icons on the otherwise-bare walls. At Saint Dionysios, the largest and sturdiest of the churches I entered, a splintered wooden doorway led me, unexpectedly, onto a flat roof crowned with a cupola and blessed with a view of the sea.

The smooth pathway leading from one church to the next dwindled to a narrow track that left my black leggings flecked with grass seeds. When the trail was interrupted by a rocky landslide, I had to pack my phone camera away to keep both hands free.

After I'd picked my course over the unsteady stones, the condition of the path improved for a while. Broad steps scattered with fallen pine needles approached a cluster of neatly maintained buildings dedicated to Saint Kyriaki, locked and shuttered, with an iron bell chained to the branch of a tree. Once I took the trail signposted for the Kastro, though, the track became treacherous again. Hand-scrawled signs warned me to take care and I watched every step, fitting my feet between grey rocks that bloomed with orange lichen as — waving a leafy twig to clear my way of spiderwebs — I climbed to the summit of Paleochora.

My breath was ragged by the time I reached the top. There, I found the remains of the citadel bathed in honeyed sunlight: the double church of Saints Dimitrios and George, and a dilapidated underground cistern that gave me pause — this was not a good place to stumble or fall.

In all my time in Paleochora, I met only a single soul, a shaggy-maned lion of a cat who greeted me when I first entered the site. I watched with trepidation as he stalked towards me, a determined glint in his yellow eyes. This wasn't my first encounter with one of Aegina's feral strays. The last had left a stinging scratch on my arm, evidence of an unprovoked skirmish at a harbourside taverna the night before. That mangy-looking feline had snatched the food from my fork without warning, and the skin from my wrist in the process. This golden-eyed boy, though, was hungry only for cuddles. His purr idled like a tractor as he pushed his head into my hand.

He waylaid me again as I left Paleochora, leaning into my body as I ran my hand over his unkempt fur. It was hard to tear myself away, but my bus to the Temple of Aphaia would pass through around 10.30 a.m. and I couldn't miss the opportunity to visit Moni Agios Nektarios first.

Countless miracles have been attributed to Saint Nektarios. He was a healer, much-loved in his lifetime and venerated after his death. He established this monastic enclave for women in 1904 and they named it Agia Triada, for the Holy Trinity. This is where he spent the last dozen years of his life.

Wrapping my shawl around my waist like a sarong and pulling on a light, hooded jacket to cover my head and shoulders, I entered the grounds through a back gate. I didn't have long to linger, but I paused for a few respectful moments in each of the monastery's chapels as I made my way down the hillside. In a neat stone mausoleum topped with a terracotta-tiled dome, the faithful pressed their ears to a marble tomb in the hope of hearing heavenly taps from within, signalling a blessing from the saint.

I hurried past the massive modern church below the nunnery, with only a glimpse through its doors, but I missed my bus anyway. With a seventy-five-minute wait until the next, and two more iconic landmarks to visit before I could call it a day, I took the easy option. I flagged down a taxi as it pulled away from the church, where it had dropped off a carload of pilgrims. The driver was happy to pick up another fare.

Ten euros and ten minutes later, I was queuing behind a group of German teenagers outside the sanctuary of a nymph-goddess who bore the distinction of being worshipped — in her manifestation as Aphaia — on Aegina alone. Her story, as is true of so many tales from the Bronze Age, can be a confronting one for women. She may have been the daughter of Zeus, but she also suffered at the hands of mortal men.

The goddess Aphaia was once a Cretan nymph named Britomartis. Writers of ancient times tell us she lived in the era of Minos, the king of Crete renowned for imprisoning the human-flesh-eating Minotaur in a labyrinth. The complex legends surrounding the birth and death of the Minotaur culminate in the horrendous betrayal of Ariadne, abandoned by the man she loved to die on a deserted island. Ariadne survived, but that was no thanks to Theseus.

Theseus may have been a particularly toxic example of Bronze Age attitudes to predatory sex, but he was far from the only one. It was a dangerous time to be a woman, and even a goddess couldn't count herself safe. When King Minos wouldn't take no for an answer, Britomartis escaped by flinging herself into the seas off Crete, where she became entangled in a fishing net.

Fisherfolk rescued the nymph from their net and brought her to Aegina, but instead of the island being the refuge she sought, she found herself again under threat of sexual assault. Her only escape was to disappear completely — and this sanctuary was built at the place where she vanished. It was here on Aegina that Britomartis became known as Aphaia, a name which means 'she who disappeared'.

The high school students were excited and noisy, but their teachers soon settled them under the shady trees skirting the archaeological site. Leaving their chatter behind, I climbed the steps to the graceful temple overlooking the Aegean Sea far below. Despite the goddess's grim backstory, my heart lifted at the summit and I thought of her vanishing as a victory. Britomartis may have been worshipped on Crete but, in all the sprawling territory of Ancient Greece, it was only on Aegina that a temple was constructed to honour the moment of her mysterious disappearance.

This sanctuary has been sacred to Aphaia for four millennia, but the current structure was built around 500 BCE, after an earlier monument was destroyed by fire. At the north-eastern edge of the hilltop plateau, a towering column topped by a crouching sphinx survived the flames, but it is long gone now. Only the base remains, alongside a hole in the ground that leads to an underground cistern. You can still walk along the stone-cut channel that fed rainwater from the temple's roof down into the cistern's gaping mouth.

It was almost noon before I realised the low stone building fifty metres away was an archaeological museum, so my peaceful hour in Aphaia's sanctuary ended with an eight-minute rush around the museum's exhibits, photographing every panel so I could read them later. I was ravenous, and eager to catch the 12.10 p.m. bus to Aegina Town and its row of tavernas and cafés overlooking the harbour.

~ ~ ~

By the time I called in to my accommodation for a bathroom break on my way to the seaside Temple of Apollo, my boots were dusty and my cheeks were flushed from the *tetarto* of white wine that came with my hard-earned lunch of grilled vegetables and halloumi. As I headed back out to find the fourth unforgettable heritage site of the day — Apollo's lone column would turn out to be part of a multilayered archaeological complex encompassing six thousand years of human habitation — I ran into Stavroula. When she heard I'd been to Paleochora, her face brightened.

'I tell everyone,' she said. 'But nobody goes.'

**Want to keep exploring the
Greek mainland and islands?**

Sign up to Sally Jane Smith's newsletter at
www.sallyjanesmith.com/newsletter
to be notified when the next story in the *Packing for Greece*
series lands on shelves,
or visit
www.linktr.ee/SallyJaneSmith
to access gorgeous photos, travel puzzles,
podcasts and more.

BOOK CLUBS

I REMEMBER FEELING SO GROWN up when I joined my first book club, all the way back in… hmmm, around the turn of the century, I think! Since then, I've belonged to a few, as I've moved from one country to another, and I've formed lasting friendships over a shared love of books.

Some clubs enjoy a structured analysis of a book, while others choose to chat freestyle. These are some optional questions to help guide a discussion of *Repacking for Greece*. Please use as many or as few of them as you please.

If scheduling allows, I'm happy to join book club gatherings via Zoom or similar — you're welcome to contact me at www.sallyjanesmith.com/contact.

If you prefer to chat without the author present, I'd still love to hear about it — and see it, too. Feel free to tag me in your group photos on social media or email me a pic.

1.   Have you travelled to Greece? Did anything about the book's setting feel familiar? Why, or why not?

2.   What was your favourite passage in the book, and why?

3.   In Chapter One, Sally described her parents as 'kind people who tried to lead good lives.' What did you think of them by the end of the story?

4.   Sally said that Nelson Mandela's release rally was 'both the most wonderful and the most dreadful day of my young life.' Based on her description, did you think it was more a positive or a negative experience?

5.   *Repacking for Greece* travels to Athens, Delphi, Corfu, Kefalonia, Nafplio, Mycenae, Epidavros, Poros, Hydra and Methana, as well as a few side trips. How many of these did you know about before reading Sally's story?

6.   What did you think of Sally's decision to climb around a locked gate in Delphi and then, by contrast, not to walk

among the archaeological remains at the Mon Repos estate on Corfu? Would you have made a different decision at either site? Why or why not?

7.   Were you surprised that Sally wasn't travelling with her partner, Adam? How would you prefer to travel: solo, in an organised tour group, or with family or friends?

8.   Had you read any of the books mentioned in *Repacking for Greece*? Did you enjoy the literary references in the story? Are there any books you would have added to a Greece-focused reading list?

9.   The book is dedicated both to Adam and to 'everyone who showed me kindness in Sri Lanka'. How did you feel about what happened after Sally's bus accident?

10. Sally has strong opinions about respectful travel — yet she unthinkingly intruded on a Greek Orthodox church service on Kefalonia. Did this affect your view of Sally as a traveller? Have you ever done something on your travels that you later regretted?

11. *Repacking for Greece* describes Sally's second trip to Greece in less than a year. If you had the same opportunities for travel, would you spend all your time in one country, as Sally did, or would you choose to explore as many countries as possible?

12. A number of legendary characters — including female figures such as Clytemnestra, Helen and Britomartis — are mentioned in the book. Which character from Ancient Greek mythology most appeals to you?

13. The Aegina chapter was set six years after the rest of the story, and was written more than five years after this book's first draft. Did you notice any changes in Sally's approach to travel or her writing voice?

14. Did you learn anything about Greece that surprised you?

15. If you could visit just one place described in *Repacking for Greece*, which would it be and why?

ACKNOWLEDGEMENTS

A PPARENTLY, I WENT ON a bit too long with my acknowledgements in *Unpacking for Greece*. Gratitude will do that. I'll keep this version a little shorter by saying that, given that I wrote the two books in tandem, pretty much everyone I thanked in the first book also contributed to the foundations of the second. I won't list all their names again, but I'm grateful to each and every one of them.

Although Book Two was already a near-final draft by the time Book One landed on shelves, it still took a lot of work to bring it to completion. Much of this work was done on Darkinyung and Guringai land on Australia's beautiful NSW Central Coast. In the early days of this manuscript, I was also privileged to participate in a residency at Varuna, The National Writers' House, which sits on Dharug and Gundungurra land in the Blue Mountains. I acknowledge and pay my respects to the traditional custodians of these lands.

My 'sisters' — Jenny Gardner, Tassin Barnard, Megan McEvoy and Shauna Bradley — were my sounding board for difficult decisions and a constant reassuring presence when I felt disheartened or overwhelmed. Beta readers Eileen Huestis, Judith Benson, Lisa Rose Wright and Valerie Poore — and Samantha Sirimanne Hyde, who gave feedback on the Sri Lanka chapter — were generous with their time and their advice. Liana Magrath assisted with maps, logo, and humorous cat videos. Wendy Brooke and Melissa Joulwan generously accepted advanced review copies of *Repacking for Greece*, and followed up with the thoughtful endorsements that grace the cover.

Not only did Kate Sclavos organise accommodation for me on Kefalonia, she once again bookended my writing journey, being both my first alpha reader and, six years later, the very last to read the manuscript before typesetting. The last, that is, apart from my sister Jenny, who — having been the first to notice a missing capital letter in my earlier book — volunteered to give this one a final read-through to spot any typos that might have slipped through the editing cracks.

Maria A. Karamitsos, an important voice in the world of Greek and Greece-focused literature, has championed my first book and given valuable advice on the second. She has introduced my work to many in the Greek-American community, and their warm welcome has awoken in me a deeper comprehension of *philoxenia*.

ACKNOWLEDGEMENTS

Writing is a solitary pursuit, yet authors are often sustained by like-minded communities of readers and writers. I am no exception. I'd particularly like to thank the Words on the Waves Writers' Festival, my new friends of CoastWrite, the wonderfully supportive Binders and We Love Memoirs groups on Facebook, and the family of writers from Limnisa. My Facebook 'word warriors' deserve a mention too. This group of friends has helped immensely over the years, especially when I've needed to assess regional language usage, word connotations and general knowledge.

The role of the professional editor in bringing a book to the literary stage is often underestimated. Carol Major, Elisabeth Chretien and Tony Reeder gave useful feedback on parts of this narrative when they were included in early drafts of *Unpacking for Greece*, and I count myself especially lucky to have worked with two highly skilled women to adapt *Repacking for Greece* into a stand-alone story. An author might be both choreographer and performer of the storytelling dance, but a good editor is the coach who stands behind them, pointing out every weakness, challenging the dancer to push their body to the limits and to reach, always, for a cleaner line.

Jacqui Brown's professional assessment of the manuscript was invaluable. She confirmed my growing belief that *Repacking for Greece* deserved its own story, and pointed out gaps that needed to be filled to make it a satisfying read.

Emily Miller came to my manuscript in its final stages, and I thank the Muses for bringing her into my writing life. Emily's copy edits curb my worst tendencies towards overly flowery prose, so I will keep this acknowledgement simple: *Repacking for Greece* is a better book because of her input.

When it came to turning the manuscript into a physical artefact, I couldn't have hoped for better partners than Andrew and Rebecca Brown from Design for Writers. It was Rebecca's patient formatting that turned the words on my screen into the pages of a real book. And I didn't think Andrew could surpass the cover he produced for *Unpacking for Greece*, yet here we are!

Everyone mentioned in *Repacking for Greece* has enriched my travels, my writing or my life, but Aruna Rajapaksa, Anne Chamila Ragavan and their families deserve the highest accolades for coming to the aid of a stranger in need. There will never be words strong enough to express my gratitude.

And Adam. This publishing journey would have been so much harder without his support. He drives me to bookstores and DIY writing retreats, accepts with good grace when I turn down lunch dates to work on edits, tolerates 3.00 a.m. wake-ups for international book club meetings, picks up more than his fair share of the housework, and is my biggest social media fan. I'm looking forward to being able to spend more time with him once this book has made it out into the world.

ACKNOWLEDGEMENTS

I said I'd keep it shorter this time, but the word count is mounting. So I'd better stop here, with a blanket acknowledgement to the countless other people who have helped me in numerous ways, not least the librarians, booksellers, book clubs, bloggers, podcasters, journalists and readers who have shown up to support the *Packing for Greece* series.

You have made this experience one of the most rewarding of my life. Thank you.

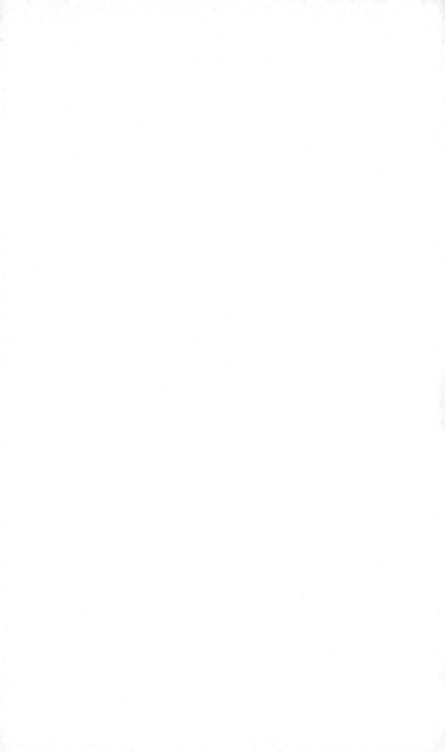

In a story told with warmth, humour and a fascination with Greece's natural and cultural heritage, Sally connects with her past, overcomes her fears and falls in love with life again, one olive at a time.

Book One in the *Packing for Greece* series travels to Athens and Meteora on the mainland; Monemvasia, Sparta and Methana on the Peloponnese Peninsula; and the islands of Santorini and Rhodes.

'A truly literary memoir — a story of tragedy, resilience and the gradual rediscovery of adventure. Sally takes you with her in every sense.'
Ned Kelly award-winning and *USA Today* best-selling author, Sulari Gentill

ABOUT THE AUTHOR

SALLY JANE SMITH HAS lived on five continents and visited thirty-three countries, but she gives credit to Greece for turning her into a writer. She has worked in museums, universities, a language institute, a residence for people with disabilities, an art gallery, a primary school and a wildlife park. She also co-hosts two book clubs and assists the organisers of a biennial book-themed convention. She is currently based in Australia.

Sally is the author of the first two books in the *Packing for Greece* series, *Unpacking for Greece: Travel in a Land of Fortresses, Fables, Ferries and Feta* and *Repacking for Greece: A Mediterranean Odyssey*. She completed a Varuna residency in 2018 and has published travel articles in *Gulf News*, *JourneyWoman* and *TripFiction*, and craft pieces in *Women's Ink!* and *Brevity Blog*. Sally's story of her great-great-grandmother's extraordinary life appears in the anthology *Itchy Feet: Tales of Travel and Adventure*. Her exploration of travel and grief is included in the *Newcastle Short Story Award Anthology 2022*.

Excerpts from the *Packing for Greece* series have been

awarded First Place Non-Fiction in the Port Writers Open Literary Competition and shortlisted in the National Writing Competition organised by the Society of Women Writers NSW. In July 2023, *Unpacking for Greece* was selected as Reading Greece Book of the Month by *Greek News Agenda*, a Greek government website.

Printed in Great Britain
by Amazon